IT'S O.K.
TO TALK ABOUT SEX
A Guide for Parents of Newborns Through Adolescence

Jane Carney Schulze and Rolf Schulze

Createspace

Library of Congress Control Number: 2001 134162
ISBN-13: 978-1463563264
ISBN-10: 1463563264

Cover design by Amara Wahaba Karuna

Illustrations by Charles H. Wallace IV,

and Amara Wahaba Karuna

Text design by Rena Wallace

2nd Edition

This publication expresses the opinions and ideas of its authors with the hope that it will provide useful information on the subjects covered. This book is sold with the understanding that the authors are not engaged in giving medical, health, psychological or any other kind of professional services. If needed, the reader should consult competent medical, health or any other professional assistance.

The authors specifically disclaim all responsibility for any liability, loss or risk, personal or otherwise, which might occur as a consequence, directly, or indirectly, of the use of and application of any of the contents of this book, which is intended only to provide suggestions and alternatives to be considered by the reader.

For our children, Bonnie, Dan, Eric, Mark and Amara
and grandchildren,
Erica, Guy Peter, Heron, Jason, Levon, Russell and Ryan
-- who deserve our best.

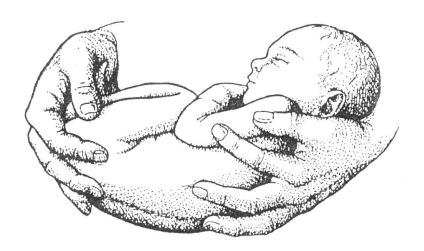

FOREWORD

Is it OK to talk about sex? Of course it is; we do it all the time. News and entertainment media, video stores and internet outlets thrive on sensationalizing sexual issues for us, making money exploiting the exotic extremes and tantalizing mysteries while muting our more mundane but intensely personal search for constructive, enriching relationships. We trade "dirty" jokes and foster gender discrimination. We may passively or actively inflame distrust and even hatred toward others whose sexual styles differ from our own. Generation after generation we have grown up to ask, "What is the world coming to?" as we deplore the continuing failure of society to respect and protect our cherished nostalgia for the "good old days" of sexual "normalcy". And as we talk, talk, talk about sex among ourselves we hope our children will remain silent: innocent and ignorant of "premature" sexual awareness.

Wrapped in our own morbid fascinations and relentless intrigues, we imagine that sexual awareness is too dangerous, too complicated for children to comprehend. It's OK for us, among ourselves, to talk about sex. But is it OK to talk about sex with our children? Parents may believe it is, may think they should, but still cop out to uncertainty and awkward avoidance. "Of course it's OK to talk with my kids about sex. But certainly not while they're little. Maybe when they're older. Maybe in junior high. But not if it lets them get sexual. You can't talk to high school kids about sex. They're already into stuff I couldn't even imagine. Don't want to talk about it!

Some thirty years ago I led a classroom discussion group in sexual issues at a local high school. The weekly seminar offered adolescent boys and girls the rare opportunity to explore ideas and concerns beyond their usual girl-only, boy-only, kids-only select circles. I was amazed at the individual diversity and the earnest candor that emerged in those sessions. Kids seemed willing to open up with each other, with a teacher and even with an outside shrink, but rarely with their parents. "My parents just won't talk about sex."

During that same period I shared with a family physician an attempt at parent-child sex education sponsored by our YMCA. We met with a self-selected group of parents and alternately with their adolescent children. The kids were open in discussing their interests and uncertainties with us. The parents were more rigid. We urged them to share with their children the beauty and pleasures of their personal sexuality. They urged us to do more to frighten their kids with the dangers of disease and impregnation. The "graduation" event, a combined parent-child discussion, was a painful exercise in evasive silence. There was no acceptable common ground. It was not OK to talk about sex.

I believe there is no less need today to try to help parents to regain the central role in transmitting positive, healthy, self-fulfilling and mutually responsible attitudes and experiences in sexual development. The stakes are even higher and the issues more pitched now than in 1968: potentially fatal illness, increasing teenage and single parenthood, gender advocacy and opposition groups vying for exposure and political representation, internet chat rooms hosting anonymous predators. Exposure is everywhere but understanding is scarce. We can never insulate our children from sexual intrigue, so we must mobilize to provide pre-emptive enlightenment and guidance.

This book, drawn from the authors' real life experience in early childhood education, sex education, parenting and grand parenting, can't put all the right words in the mouths of all parents, nor can it sensitize us to every potential question from the mouths of babes. But it can, and does, try. Against the deafening cacophony of public commotion it offers a thoughtful, authoritative guide to the gentle, formative power of confident, confiding parent-child communication.

Roland C. Summit, M.D.   November 4, 2001

ROLAND C. SUMMIT, M.D.

Dr. Summit retired in 1997 after developing a remarkable 31-year career as the community psychiatrist of Los Angeles County Harbor-UCLA Medical Center in Torrance, California. Consultation with schools, various child and family service agencies and especially with self-help groups gave him an unprecedented, inside view of the dynamics of child abuse, including multigenerational cycles of dysfunctional child rearing. He is acknowledged as the international pioneer in defining the professionally underrated frequency and seriousness of sexual abuse of children. His 1983 Child Sexual Abuse Accommodation Syndrome has been endorsed by fellow specialists as the single most influential paper in the field of child sexual abuse. Involved as he has been in the tragic misuse of sexual experience in child development, he has been dedicated equally to explore the vital importance of parents modeling and actively teaching the ideals of developmentally appropriate, love-enhancing sexuality. Dr. Summit and Jo, his wife of 44 years, have four children and three grandchildren.

IT'S OKAY TO TALK ABOUT SEX
A Guide for Parents of Newborns through Adolescence

TABLE OF CONTENTS

INTRODUCTION

*"The end and aim of sex education is
developing one's fullest capacity for love."*
Dorothy Baruch (1959)

The moment may come without warning. Your small child looks up with a question, "What does sex mean?" or "Where do babies come from?" Why, we think, didn't they ask an easy one like, "Where's God?" or "Why is the sky blue?" We know that to say, "Ask your grandma," or "You'll understand when you get older," is a cop out. The child is waiting for an answer. Your answer can be very important for you and your child. But talking to our children about sex doesn't have to be frightening. As parents, grandparents, or teachers we are the most important educators our children will ever have. We are responsible for helping them grow into happy, mature adults. We can give them good answers that stay with them long after such questioning moments are gone.

Why do many of us feel a nagging anxiety and uncertainty when the "S" word comes up? Why don't the words come easily like they do when the child asks, "Why do I have to eat my vegetables?" Memories of our childhood feelings come flooding in. Memories of our parents, grandparents and teachers struggling for the right words when we asked questions about sex. Or maybe we never asked because we picked up early silent signals from grown-ups. "Don't ask me about the 'S' word. I can't handle it."

Our children get mixed signals every day. Sexual behavior is seen in most movies and TV. Children can find some form of "sex" on every news stand. Many books describe every detail of how the body looks and works, yet explaining it to a child so they can understand, or to a teenager who wants to know more than the books tell them, is a tough job. It's also an opportunity we can't afford to miss. Our children count on us to answer their questions. Who else can they trust to answer them honestly?

This book came to life because many of our college students and other prospective parents asked for it. Sometime, during each semester, as soon as our students are seated and, hopefully, attentive, we ask, "How many of you had helpful sex education at home or in your schools?" Three or four students out of fifty usually raise their hands. We continue on. "Where did you find out about sex?" A brave soul raises her hand. "I was lucky. I had an older sister who told me the basics. But one day she sort of threw a condom my way, looked embarrassed and said, 'Be sure the guy wears this.' I was 13 and didn't know anything. I wouldn't have dared ask Mom or Dad!" Another student volunteered that his parent had left books about adolescent development on the coffee table but no one seemed to be able to discuss them.

A student in the back of the room got a laugh when he said he always seemed to know more than his parents about sexual subjects. He said he learned about sex from his buddies. Gradually, the students relax as the discussion goes on, but their frustration tells us something important. Can we afford to let our children grow into adulthood, uncertain, scared, and ignorant about their growing bodies, their sexual feelings, and the chance that they may have or cause an unwanted pregnancy, or contract a life-threatening disease? We love them far too much for that. Of course, we want to do the right thing for our children. But since children don't come with instruction booklets, we may have a hard time trying to keep a step ahead of them in this most important job called child rearing.

"Wash behind your ears, eat your yummy carrots, and please say 'thank you'" comes easily to us as parents. That's what our Mom and Dad, or Granny said to us. But let the discussion veer into the direction of male-female love relationships, intimacy and responsible sex, and our conversation sputters and often stops.

If our parents had no words to explain sexuality to us, where do we find the words? When our teachers pretended not to hear a four-year old preschooler ask, "Where do babies come from?" we felt their embarrassment. How can we overcome such embarrassment and break through that kind of silence with children? Our children and our students are watching us closely even though they would never admit it. They desperately want and need guidance. You and I have been elected. We are their guides. It's exciting and at the same time, it can be scary to be given such responsibility.

This book is about helping you do a better job of answering your child's healthy curiosity about sex and sexual development. It is also about understanding that we communicate differently with babies and young children than we do with our preteens and teens. Young ones learn slowly about their sexuality and we know to take time and to have patience as we guide them. Children come into the world feeling good about their bodies. We want them always to feel that way. Being parents and grandparents, we have also been through difficult moments when we asked ourselves, "What should we tell them and at what age?" "How honest should we be?" "What if they ask before I'm ready with good answers?" "What if we tell them too much, will they get in trouble?" Or "What if they don't ask me anything about sex?" There are times when we say things we wish we hadn't said or we leave things out that we have to add later on. Sometimes we mistakenly give out wrong information. Gratefully, we have discovered that children and students forgive us our mistakes and teach us better ways to communicate.

The first chapter discusses some effective ways to communicate with our children on any subject, not just sex. If we want our children to listen and respect us, it's important for us to communicate in ways that get their attention and make a positive impression.

There are successful ways to help children understand and feel good about their growing bodies and their sexuality. We hope this book helps you feel more confident and comfortable as you guide your child through the all-important area of sexual self-understanding. We would never withhold good nutrition or medical help from our child. Neither should we withhold good sex education. When your child can talk easily with you about sex, you have given him or her a precious gift for which they will be grateful all their lives. We hope this book helps make your job of parenting a little easier and your child's job of growing up as joyful as it is meant to be.

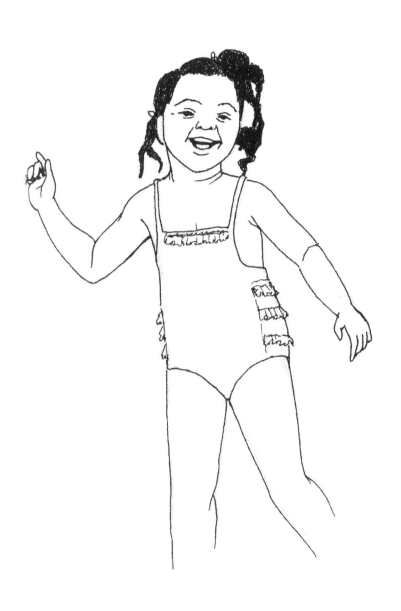

CHAPTER 1

LET'S TALK, O.K.??

Communication is the Foundation for Building Trust with Your Child from Birth On

We would all like to talk to our children about the facts of life with a minimum of awkwardness and embarrassment. Try doing it when they are just old enough to understand a few simple words. Remember, they began life with a healthy feeling about their body and see all parts of themselves as natural.

They aren't going to feel shy, even if we do. They will always notice our attitudes, however, and fortunately, we don't have to wait until they are able to understand our words for us to begin sharing and letting them know that we are comfortable with all of their body. Newborns are very sensitive to gentle voices and touching (Berk, 2002). The first day of our baby's life is the first day learning begins about their sexuality as they are gently touched, cuddled and rocked. Whether you are aware of it or not, today is the best time to start your child's sex education by giving the closeness and loving attention they require to be healthy.

Since babies are not born with fear and anxiety about sex, it seems reasonable to think that they have a relaxed attitude about this whole subject and do not understand what the big fuss is about. We hope that they are getting the message that food, closeness and touch are special feelings that they like. So we hug them, pat them, give gentle massages and play all kinds of games to get them to smile and giggle.

Brain research shows that infants need frequent and gentle touching (Prescott, 1975) and social stimulation. Holding, stroking and patting your baby assists in the normal growth of the nervous system and brain patterns and is basic to communication and a vital part of building trust. Babies need and like to be touched. It stimulates the growth of their brain pathways and helps in their development (Papalia & Olds, 1996).

Children crave touch, eye contact, and other kinds of attention. They let us know when and how much they need. If we watch them closely, we

1

can notice their signals. The more these needs are met, the happier and healthier babies and children will be and the more secure and comfortable they will be with their sexuality as they grow.

This trust building process is universal across all cultures. For example, Dr. Brock Chisolm, past director of the U.N.'s World Health Organization tells of the time he visited a maternity ward in India. The nurses were apologetic about the primitive conditions there. Dr. Chisolm disagreed. It was a very up-to-date ward, he told them. At the end of each mother's bed, there was a little hammock for the baby. When the baby cried the mother rocked the hammock with her toe or picked up the child to comfort or feed it. The need of those babies for closeness was being met from birth on, they were learning to trust their mothers and the world outside the womb.

Children usually let us know when they want to be touched. Some babies want to be held every waking hour. No, it does not spoil them (Spock, 1998), even though you're sure you will never get the time to clean house again. Another baby, in the same family, can sleep for four or five hours, wake up to eat for 20 minutes and go back to sleep (ours did).

Babies come with their own unwritten instructions and we know we've succeeded by the way their bodies suddenly calm down and snuggle up to us, or by the grin we get for doing it right. Once their needs are taken care of, they settle down to sleep or play happily with whatever is available. When they wake up they are ready to explore, touch, taste and poke at everything in their path including their own bodies. Eventually they will also touch their sexual organs, whether we are around or not. When they are bored with those parts they will probably grab a toe to chew.

Before we knew better, when a parent, a relative or a babysitter saw the baby touching their sexual parts, the all too common reaction was, at best, to quickly direct them to a toy or, at worst, to slap their hand and say, "No, dirty!" And what might the child be learning? "What's going on?" What felt so good to them seems bad. "My special person inflicts pain on me just for touching there. I must be bad and that feeling I liked must also be bad." That realization can be the beginning of serious personality and/or sexual problems. This experience of punishment can become part of a body memory, which leaves the grown child with a sense of fear and guilt whenever they become involved in sex (Erickson, 1963).

2

A therapist was once asked by a young mother about the best age to start educating her child about sexuality. He responded by asking, "What's your child's age?" "Six years old," she replied. The therapist answered, "I hope you started six years ago."

We know that being comfortable with our bodies starts at birth with touching and closeness. But what do we do when children are old enough to talk to us about it? If we have known how to build trust with a child during the early years, they will want to confide in us and, hopefully ask us questions just as they ask about all other subjects.

It is a special moment when your child or grandchild comes to you with questions concerning sexual matters. It means they trust you to give them the best and the most truthful answers you can give. This is the time to let them know that you appreciate and welcome such questions so the child knows its O.K. to talk.

When you want a child to eat nutritious food you do not try to force-feed them peas and carrots if their mouths are clamped shut. Instead, you smack your lips and taste the mashed carrots with great enthusiasm, then offer the spoon with a smile, inviting the child to do the same. If you are refused, you know to try later.

It is the same with sexual matters. Start in their early years and introduce the subject honestly in a relaxed way. Bring up the subject naturally as you talk with the child. They will ask for more when they are ready and then you will talk with them about their concerns.

If you want to make sure that your child's curiosity about human sexuality gets satisfied, here are some ways to introduce the subject.

1. Be alert to even small opportunities. Pregnant animals in the neighborhood offer an opportunity to pay a visit to the new kittens, puppies or hamsters.

Our grandchild prefers snakes! Birds in nests are great, too. Be sure you comb the bookstores for baby animal books (See References). Then fill in the explanations your child seems to want. *Give simple and truthful answers the child can understand.*

2. Visit a newborn baby. If possible, let your child feel the baby move before it is born. Have books with lots of simple pictures to help explain birth at the level the child can understand. You'll know it's a sure sign of boredom when your child starts to wiggle, look elsewhere, or takes the book out of your hand and closes it.

3. <u>Be careful not to push any subject too hard</u>. No one likes a pushy salesperson. You may have noticed that the more anxious we are to get our point across, the more likely our audience is to back off. This definitely includes children.

4. <u>Make Visual Material Available with Sensitivity</u>. Even while offering as much information or discussion as they are willing to digest, sometimes showing a more advanced book is all right if you show only the pictures and make up the words. If you are comfortable with the subject and like the book, chances are the child will also like it.

Even if your toddler or preschooler wiggles away after a brief time, do not be discouraged. The information has, no doubt, begun to filter into their memory banks and even more importantly, you are relaxed. That feeling of "I'm enjoying my time with you" will be remembered. There will be a next time to look forward to.

5. <u>Watch for Spontaneously Occurring Opportunities</u>. That next time might be at the bath hour or when you are diapering an older child's baby brother, sister or cousin.

"What's that?" a three-year old may ask when her new baby brother is first diapered. It is easy enough for you to say, "That's his penis…his tinkle or urine (or whatever your family says) comes out there. That's different from yours, isn't it?" You may get a nod of agreement and notice that your daughter is undressing so she can see how different she really is. She may be resourceful enough to find a mirror to help.

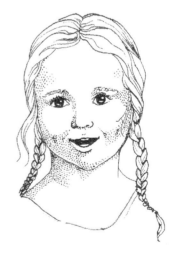

Answer her questions and be supportive of her attempts to find out what she looks like. As soon as she is satisfied about what she is interested in, she will no doubt, jump up and ask for a snack or want to go out and play. You can breathe a sigh of relief. Her ongoing sex education is continuing to be a positive experience.

4

You have played an important part in developing her healthy attitude about her body. If she wants to ask more questions (as in the above example), and you continue to answer as honestly as possible, you are likely to find that this communication will get easier as time goes by. Your child will want to keep asking questions. Remember, first learning is the most powerful learning and remains in the child's memory for a long time.

GUIDELINES FOR GOOD COMMUNICATION

What are the main guidelines for good listening to help us communicate better? Professionals, such as Haim Ginott (1969) and Thomas Gordon (1970) have written about the importance of "active listening." These basic guidelines are as follows:

1. Listen with all your attention, and with good eye contact. Think about the people you most like to talk with. Chances are they are good listeners. When someone gives us their full attention they are saying to us, "You are important to me and I respect you and really want to listen to you."

2. Respond with listening words like, "Oh, I see," or "Mmm."

3. Try to describe the child's feelings as if you were guessing at them. For example, "It seems to me you're feeling sad, or scared."

4. Describe the child's wishes and hopes. "I wish you could have a new bike, too, but we can't get it now because…." At least the child knows you are trying to understand his feelings. Resist the temptation to solve the problem for the child. You could ask, "I wonder what could be done about that?" and watch the child's facial expression, giving her time to think it through if she is ready.

Avoid blaming, judging, name calling, or teasing. That takes unfair advantage of children who can't defend themselves. That kind of behavior never solves problems at any age. Try to express your feelings by telling them how you feel, using the "**I**" word ("I feel that… or, "I want…"). Avoid the negative "**You** did it!" attitude. This way, the child is being respected and listened to. At the same time, the child is not getting everything she wants, when you feel its not good for her. So you set limits and hold your ground (see section on Discipline). Even with the best discipline techniques, children do not always take our word as the final one. They test us constantly by asking, demanding, crying, maybe even throwing a tantrum, to try to get what they want at the

5

moment. This is their way of finding out how far they can go. After all, no one gave them an Instruction Booklet on Life either. The way we react to this kind of noisy behavior is basic to building trust with a child and setting firm limits. Limit setting can be one of our toughest tasks. If we do it well, our children benefit from our strength all their lives and we will enjoy our parenting.

BUILDING TRUST: The First Step to Good Communication

What is this thing called "Good Communication?" This phrase is tossed about as the answer to all parent-child problems. We would like to be able to communicate well with our children from their first days. Even if you have older children, and your communication with them is not what you would like, keep trying. It's never too late to do a better job of communicating.

Here are some guidelines:

1. <u>Good Communication is Not One-Sided</u>. If you find yourself talking excitedly into a silent blank expression and glazed-over eyes, even if the head in front of you is nodding up and down, that's probably not good communication.

2. <u>Good Communication Depends on Mutual Trust</u>. Trust starts building on Day One of any relationship. For instance, a one-month-old baby has a need that is very important to him or her, such as hunger. The grown up observes the need and hears the cry, then fills the need satisfactorily. Suddenly, trust blossoms between the two (Erickson, 1963). What has happened here? The grown-up has shown respect for the child's need. Once the child's needs are met, the child then begins the process of learning that the world is a safe and good place with his family. Later, the child will be able to understand how to respond to other's needs, as he grows older. Good communication is developing. If, for some reason, you have to start building trust when the child is older, it is still possible. Just follow the same guidelines discussed in these pages, beginning as soon as possible. Let the child know you are sorry that things were not better in the past, but that the two of you are starting out new. As long as you speak honestly, the child will be more likely to respond positively when ready.

A young child is too inexperienced to try to fool or lie to the grown-up. A child's feelings are right out in front for the entire world to see, unless they have been frightened into hiding them (Summit, 1992). The grown-up's actions are what the child will watch. As the grown-up earns the child's trust, the child keeps returning for attention and help. The child's return to the adult for help is the ultimate compliment.

To be worthy of the child's trust, be careful to promise only what you are quite sure you can deliver. This includes rewards as well as other kinds of discipline. If you have promised a bedtime story or payment of earned allowance on Saturday, be sure you follow through. If you said "No TV unless you pick up your toys," then keep your word. If circumstances cause you to have to make a change, an explanation or an apology is in order. Children love apologies from grown-ups because, too often, the child seems to be the one making the mistakes. Children can handle disappointments and surprises if they can be helped to understand what is really happening.

3. <u>Sometimes Trust is Hard to Build</u>. There are circumstances in a child's life when they become afraid to trust adults and will try to hide their feelings as best they can. This behavior often occurs when children have been victims of child sexual abuse and have been frightened into remaining silent. It is very important that we be aware of what happens to a child when close adults ignore, or tune out; leaving a child to hide their pain. The Child Sexual Abuse Accommodation Syndrome (CSAAS) has been defined by Roland Summit, M.D. (1983,1990) after many years of observing children who were unable to reveal sexual abuse they had endured in silence. It is important to be aware of the following five factors of the CSAAS, all, or part of which may be found with children who have been abused:

(1)   "Secrecy" by the child and the abuser, often accompanied by threats from the adult.

(2)   The child's sense of "Helplessness" in not being able to stop the abuse.

(3)   The child's sense of "Entrapment and Accommodation." Feeling there is no way out, the child attempts to protect the secret and to adjust without complaint to continuing abuse. Child victims wish that a loving, protective parent would "just know" and rescue them. Failing that, they tend to feel they are bad and unworthy of love. Their search for some kind of relief from emotional pain may lead to substance abuse, delinquent behavior, sexual misconduct and/or a way of dissociating them from reality so they can escape into imaginary safe places with magical, reassuring companions.

(4)   A child's "Delayed, Conflicted or Unconvincing Disclosure" if they do try to talk about the abuse (most victims never tell). Because they

7

didn't tell at first, and especially because the abuser is likely to be someone known an trusted by the family, even the most caring adults find it hard to believe the child in the face of reassuring denial by the accused. Parents may avoid involving the authorities. If it does become a criminal matter, the child's conflicted testimony may be discredited by attorneys for the accused.

(5)   Finally, "Retraction" by the child. The skeptical and punishing response of the adult world drives the child back to the misguided but familiar security of secrecy and accommodation, arguing convincingly that they lied about the abuse. All too often, parents are more comfortable dismissing the child as a liar than viewing a trusted adult as a child molester.

Children who are trapped in sexual abuse need compassionate, professional intervention to assist parents in giving the child essential love and comfort while the abuse is investigated. Crisis counseling for child and parents can allow healing and life enrichment rather than the damaging long-term burden of unresolved abuse.

4. <u>Good Communication Isn't Just About Talking</u>. Children not only need food, shelter and clothing to survive. They need attention from the first day. Communication begins when they look into our eyes and coo or fuss for food and we coo back. Later we may ask, "Milk or juice?" and help them suck a nipple or sip from a cup. Have you noticed how a toddler glances at a parent before trying some new, daring maneuver, like holding onto a familiar knee before moving to a nearby chair? If the parent looks into the child's eyes, smiles, and maybe nods, that translates to the child as "Go for it, good for you." The child may move away a few inches, holding on to a nearby chair. Soon back with the parent, the whole movement is repeated until the child is able to move farther beyond the parent and play with others. Unless the parent pays that kind of quality attention and is patient as the child practices separating, the child is likely to whine and cling over a much longer period. If a parent acts impatient and pushes the child away, successful separation is not made (Papalia and Olds, 1996). When we give a child what they really need, they tend to move on to the next task while trusting us to be there for them, if we are needed.

5. <u>Good Communication Doesn't Lead to Spoiling Your Child</u>. Knowing when to fill your child's real need can be a tricky decision. If our grandparents were listening, they might scold us for trying to "spoil" the younger generation with talk of filling emotional needs. It turns out to be just the opposite. We are <u>really</u> spoiled when we don't get our real needs met. When strong needs are ignored, hurt and angry feelings and fears of abandonment keep us from being cooperative. We then have trouble listening to the wise words of those who really want to help us. Words and actions that can help a child trust a parent must be built slowly, day-by-day. The bond strengthens and the child learns that the parent will be there to fill basic needs. It must feel wonderfully secure to children when they can come back for more of the same consistent care. Their parents may offer a smile and eye contact, a warm lap, a hug, or a verbal, "good job." That is often enough. Trust is there, growing through the years. So that when children talk about their bodies, the bodies of others, and about sex, they will want to talk to their parents first. As long as we parents are around to listen, respond, and show affection, our children will continue to ask for guidance at home, not on the street. The streets for them, is a last resort.

6. <u>Good Communication is Also Watching and Listening</u>.

New parents and teachers wonder how they can be successful models for children when there is so much they need to learn. They ask questions like:

- What if I choose the wrong childcare?
- Am I giving too much or too little attention to my child?
- When should I say "no"?
- What do I do if my child ignores the "no"?

These are tricky questions and we do not always have time to look up the answers in a book. Books are great resources, but we first need to watch the child and pick up his signals. Try to become an expert child watcher. You may even be able to come up with a plan to observe your child without being noticed, while either a babysitter is helping or a teacher lets you sit quietly in a corner. We know all children react a little differently when parents are not on the scene. We can learn a lot about that child by watching and even taking some notes. We can often see the kind of reactions that we might not notice at home. An aggressive child at home may show shyness at school because they are afraid to communicate with other children. Or a child who is very quiet and obedient at home may dominate her friends at school. The teacher, school counselor and family, may be able to help pinpoint the problems, so they can work on solutions together. Even if you do not see yourself as an expert on children, you **are** the primary expert on your child's likes and dislikes. You understand that the little turned-down lip means, "Get me out of here," or "I've taken all of this I can." You know that those first little baby noises are subtle hints that hunger is approaching and your newborn is saying, "Get the food fast, Mom, I can't hold out much longer."

Young children come to us, it seems, believing that they are the center of their universe. For a while, we eagerly buy into it because they are ours and are so cute! The child development researcher, Urie Bronfenbrenner said in a 1989 speech to the United Nations that you have to be "crazy about your kid" to parent successfully. However, somewhere in the early toddler years parent patience can wear thin. We may still be "crazy about the kid," but we are forced into the role of helping our child learn the realities of personal responsibility, or face the consequences. We want them to learn to solve their problems as openly and honestly as possible while being respectful and loving. If we are successful in teaching self-responsibility to our young ones, family life and the child's experience as a human being can be truly beautiful.

7. Children Want Us To Talk With Them When THEY Are Ready to Listen. Any of us who have parented teenagers may raise an eyebrow on this one. But it is true. Children not only want our attention through praise, fun and other goodies, they really want us to talk to them and be with them. A child's world can be confusing and scary even with the best of care. They depend on us to help them sort it out and find good solutions for their fears and anger. If we are silent or absent, they will have to turn elsewhere, desperate for some kind of model.

As we have interviewed, parented and "step-parented" children of all ages, one of the biggest lessons we have learned from them sounds something like this:

"Please keep talking and listening to us even when we refuse to answer, or when we call you names, or yell at you. Please keep talking to us. Be interested in us. Don't just hear angry words or ask us questions to scold us. Hear our pain, too. Let us watch you as good models. Tell us when you make mistakes, too, so we can learn from them, and you won't seem so far away and perfect to us. Show us a safe path by your steady, wise actions. Your actions teach us everything. Then we will hear your words. We may try a dangerous path sometimes, but if you are always there waiting for us and loving us, we are likely to come back to you. We will always remember and someday you'll be glad you stood by us, loving and strong."

8. <u>You Can't Fool A Kid. Be Honest.</u> They'll call us on it sooner or later. If real trust is built on good communication, then the foundation is built on honesty. A little child may give the impression that they buy your story about the "Stork brings the baby" or "Mom or Dad aren't going out, so go to sleep." But some way, somehow, when they find out, you get demoted a notch or so on their internal trust index.

Why is it important to be such honest parents? College students tell us that hypocrisy was one big reason they lost respect for their parents or family members. "Do as I say, not as I do," will not get the job done. Young people would rather hear an apology for a parent's poor judgment or mistake, as they watch us make the necessary corrections, than to see us try to excuse our way out. With our honest apology, our child's respect for us remains intact.

9. <u>Parents Also Have Rights.</u> Communicate self-respect by treating yourself fairly and your child then learns to respect you. As they are respected and valued by those closest to them, they will value themselves and respect others. We start here with the hope that you, as a parent, already like and respect yourself. If that thought gives you problems, there are many ways to look for help (see Appendix on Support Sources).

We know of permissive parents who never learned where to draw the line on rules for their children, even in the areas of safety and health. Their children were miserable. Sometimes these parents are afraid they will lose their child's affection. Maybe the memories of their own childhood pain come back to stop them from using firm discipline. To do good parenting we have no choice but to set some limits at critical times and stick with them as long as they seem to be working well (see Chapter 2).

For example, it seems that happy, energetic children may want to talk to us constantly, during every waking hour. At some interval, you will, no doubt, be involved in a task, or an emergency, that can't be set aside, no matter how much you love your child. You then may have to say in your friendly, but firm voice, "I know that what you have to tell me is very important. Hold on for a minute, until after this phone call, and I'll be able to listen carefully." Then, remember to do just as you said. If a child has been asked to wait until later to talk, try writing a memo to yourself, and put it in plain sight so you won't forget to follow up. Your child will be impressed that you are serious about scheduling time for the two of you.

Communication with our child starts in the cradle. When we are responsive to our child's needs, trust is built between us. As our children reach the toddler and preschool years, that trust is further strengthened when we set consistent and logical limits with love for their safety, health and happiness.

We then know that we have laid the foundation for healthy communication that will allow them to successfully reach out into the world and discover their dreams. And with any luck, they will return to us as adults and want to call us "friend."

MORE TIPS FOR PARENTS

1. Babies never have to wait for food or warmth and comfort in their mother's womb, so it's wise to try to meet those needs after birth as quickly as possible, so babies aren't forced to cry hard before being fed or held.

2. Let babies cuddle with you in your bed as much as possible. Parents have to decide if they want their babies to sleep with them. In many cases, parents report that it works just fine with no problems developing later on (Berk, 1996).

3. Hold the baby when it seems to calm and comfort her. It's scary to be all alone in a cold and isolated crib.

4. Stroke the baby gently, or give pats on the back. Gentle massage will be welcomed by most babies. All that touching really does stimulate brain development.

5. Hum to the baby as you rock him. Music is soothing and all babies love it. Our grandson especially liked American Indian chants.

6. As babies develop, play games with them. They like to have you put your head on their tummies so they can touch your hair as you rub your cheek on them. You are usually rewarded with smiles and giggles.

7. There are many ways to touch babies to show them your love. Always watch their facial expressions to be sure they show that they like what you're doing. Stop right away if they show resistance. As long as their faces look happy and their bodies are not tense, you're doing fine. They can usually go on playing longer than you can.

8. When you first notice your child exploring and touching his or her sexual parts, do not react in an abrupt, shocked, or upset way. If they had decided to touch their heads, you'd behave normally, right? Children are not aware of our learned fears about sex. To them, every part of their body is to be explored, enjoyed, and accepted. We are sexual, sensual creatures and need to accept all parts of us as good, if we are to grow up healthy and happy. Of course, there are rules about our behaviors in polite society. As the child grows up, we can explain what behavior is OK at home, but not in public.

9. Just as you teach your child the names of various parts of her body, you decide what you want them to call their sexual parts. You can say "nipple" or "penis" or "vulva or vagina," if the child is touching those parts, and looking questioningly at you. Each family has their own pet names and they are all fine, as long as you are consistent. Words that respect the child without poking fun, or showing disrespect, always work best.

10. When children ask questions about sex, answer as honestly and naturally as you can, so they can understand you. Relax, look at them and smile. You'll get through it and you'll be proud of yourself.

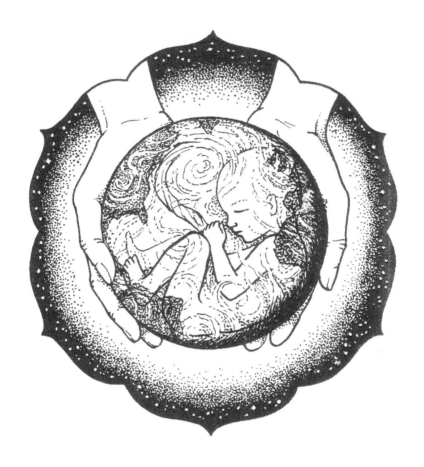

CHAPTER 2

SETTING LIMITS

One of the great shocks in store for us, early in life, is the discovery that we are not the empress or emperor of our world. If our parents did their job well, our needs as infants were satisfied. So we might think, why can't it go on like this forever? Some parents actually try catering to their child's every whim, with disastrous results for all concerned. Along with love, food and freedom, our children must experience the frustration of not always getting what they want the moment they want it. A wise parent plans for this reality and helps their child cope. We might say:

"I know you want that cookie right now. But it's time to eat carrot sticks. Cookies come later. Please put the cookie back." If you are ignored, you might then say, "I will help you put it back." Proceed to move the child's hand and the cookie back to its original spot. The cookie may end up in crumbles, but it will get back on the plate and your limit has been successfully carried out. Action is the key, once the words of explanation have been given.

Many parents and educators use a method called "problem solving" to help with the limit-setting process. Reynolds (1996) says, "The goal of problem solving is simple. It helps children learn to solve problems in a respectful, satisfying way, without fear of domination. It builds self-esteem and self-reliance." With problem solving, the child has an opportunity to talk about their needs and feelings and so does the parent. Then, hopefully, a compromise can be reached. If not, the parent must step in and make a decision, then set a limit in the family's best interest.

Our world is full of rules and laws, natural and people-made. The beauty of a child's learning is that they cope better with reality than with fantasy or dishonesty. They have trouble with inconsistent or non-existent rules. That's scary for them. Think about the adult world. Suppose that every time we approached an intersection in our automobile, we were expected to guess what the traffic rules are for that day. We'd be frustrated and miserable. The child may feel that way at home without firm rules.

We want our child to be likeable and to like him or herself. No one enjoys having a child around them who doesn't understand rules like respecting others and staying out of serious trouble. Kids who never learned to follow rules, cause themselves and others major problems. For example, when children run into the street in front of a car, or touch a flame on a stove, not only does the child suffer, but so does the family and community. Since we love our children, and have no desire for anyone to suffer, it is our job to keep them out of the street and away from harm. Other limit setting is no different. We, as parents, are here to teach and model the rules for the family, the community, and our country, so that our children will become likeable and law-abiding human beings.

BE CLEAR ABOUT THE RULES YOU DECIDE TO ENFORCE, NO MATTER WHAT!

1. Sit down with your family and make a list of the most important rules or limits you believe to be necessary for the safety, peace, and well-being of your child and family. Remember to consider your feelings when making this list. Your child needs your honest reactions to his behavior, or the limit setting won't have a chance of succeeding. With older children, ask for their ideas about the list of rules the family is creating and discuss them together. Just remember, you have the final word.

2. Include only the most important limits on your list. A child can only absorb a few rules at a time in the best of circumstances. After that, they may stop cooperating. Once the first rules are understood and obeyed thank your child for cooperating. Remember that safety, health, and respect for others, are top priority items. Consider putting clean rooms, the color of a school outfit, or whether grandma gets a hug, way down on your list of priorities in most cases.

3. Try to stay calm but firm as you set down your rules for the child. State the rules in a simple, unhurried way, using the words your child can best understand. Imagine yourself for a moment as a short two-year-old, looking high up at a grown-up, who is talking fast in words you cannot understand. No wonder we adults are sometimes ignored.

4. Keep in mind the happy thought that you are actually doing your child a favor when you set firm limits and stick with them. This may be hard to believe as your child wails, "You're mean, I don't like you!" in a supermarket, but stick to your limits. You may never

16

hear your child utter the words, "Thank you, my parent, for disciplining me," but the underlying truth is there, limits must be set. Since the child enters the world with only their own inner compass working, they start from scratch in discovering the needs, wants, and realities of the other humans around them. What better humans than their parents to guide them through rough waters until they are old enough to sail in the open sea? If we as parents don't help them, who will be kind and caring enough to take the time to guide them? Our police, social workers, teachers, and religious leaders do not have the time for all who need help, and the government has not been able to find sufficient funds either.

5. <u>Set realistic limits</u>. It is especially hard for us as parents to know how to set realistic limits and make them stick. Since only in the last few years has the word spread on how to discipline successfully, we parents were often the victims of poor discipline patterns by our own parents. Perhaps some were too permissive and let us do just about what we wanted, and still others were too harsh.

There are parents who say" I can't do a thing with this child. She runs wild at home, but as soon as she goes to my friend's house, she's a little angel." How can this be? Most likely, the friend lets the child know just what is expected of her in that house. She also clearly explains the consequences when the rules are broken and then does what she promised she would do. For example, she might say, "We take turns with these toys, and if you don't want to share, you can play in another room for a while. You have toys that are just for you if you don't feel like sharing, but these are the ones we share." Permissive parents may be afraid to discipline perhaps because their own history of harsh discipline scared them and they want to stay "friends" with their child. If parents guide their children well, then genuine friendship will follow. Other parents may take what they think is the easy way out, rather than put in the effort needed to stick with limit setting. Setting limits is a difficult and time consuming job. Whatever the reason, being overly permissive, or being an absent parent, causes many difficulties in setting goals and keeping commitments. Their children may turn to drugs and early sexual relationships to try to forget their feelings of abandonment.

Another barrier to good communication are parents who learned to be abusive to their own children from their parents. These parents take out their anger on their children by screaming, yelling, hitting, or worse. We hear reports of abuse on a daily basis. Subtle abuse rarely makes the headlines but it is just as devastating to the child. Research confirms that

17

abuses of all kinds occur when parents are mindlessly repeating the treatment they received and/or are ignorant of the principles of good child development. These parents need help! (Berns, 1997).

The main point to be made here is that children do not learn better ways of behaving by being yelled at and hit. The brain learns better in an atmosphere low in anxiety (Hendrick, 1990). Violent, dominating, harsh emotions cause a child to be afraid. They may lash out or withdraw, neither of which helps in long term learning. That's why smart teachers know children won't learn arithmetic with a paddle held over them. So, remember to stay calm, while allowing the child to talk about her feelings. Stick with the limits you have set. This way, the child will know that her side of the issue has at least been heard. Then the child is more likely to be willing to accept your limits. If the rules and limits are reasonable and understandable, the child will usually cooperate. The old idea of "Do it because I say so," sounds easy, but is not effective in getting long lasting cooperation from a child.

DECIDING ON LIMITS

You can talk to children about setting rules or limits. Let them help you decide on the right ones for your household. You may be happily surprised at the bright ideas they suggest. If this kind of decision making is used in their early years, they will probably work out their problems with you in their teenage years as well (Reynolds, 1996). To begin, you might say, "Let's talk about rules and decide why we need them. Then we can decide what to do if the rules get broken." It helps to write down your rules and put them on the wall where you can all see them. The following are some examples of good rules for setting limits and disciplining children without abusive punishment.

1. <u>Set the limit firmly</u>. "I can't let you hit Tommy," or, "No playing outside after dark."

2. <u>Let the child know you understand his/her feelings</u>. "You really would like that bike, wouldn't you? It's really hard to wait."

3. <u>Give the reason for the limit</u>. "It hurts Tommy when you hit" or, "It's not safe to be outside without a grown up," or, " It's time to get ready for bed."

4. <u>Offer an alternative</u>. The child might help you choose one. "You can ask Tommy for the next turn on the bike" or, "You can play with your friend in the morning instead of tonight."

5. <u>Follow through on the limits you set with consistency</u>. Do what you said you were going to do if the child ignores the limit. Take action! If the child keeps hitting, firmly lead him away from Tommy and the bike and say, "You seem to want that bike a lot, but you will have to come over here and think about it until you can tell Tommy what you want, and wait for the next turn". In other words, **stop the action** until the problem is solved and all involved have had a chance to cooperate.

Be consistent! If you set a limit, stick with it, no matter how long it takes. If you have to leave for some reason, tell the person who is taking your place about the rule you have made. Children get the message quickly, but will try to wait you out and hope you'll forget. If you neglect to follow through, they will learn that they can do what they want, because you're not serious. If you are consistent, the next time you make a rule, they are more likely to follow that rule.

Parents who use this method to discipline their children find that their children are more likely to cooperate throughout their childhood. These children have a chance to say how they feel and what they want. At the same time, they know that their parents are in charge, and the whole family can feel more secure.

Children need to be able to count on us to do what we say we're going to do. The world looks complicated and confusing to them, especially if they can't trust an adult. That's why we have to be sure we make rules that are reasonable and can be enforced. Threatening to "ground you in your room for the rest of your life" might make us chuckle, but will only make you feel foolish when you have to let your teenager out for dinner. A better model is the parent who says "No" to TV unless the child picks up his toys in the living room that are being tripped over. You'll have to guard the "On" button until the chore is done. If your child complains or cries, stay steadfast and don't weaken. If your child is really a hold-out, and bedtime comes, you can remind him that there is always tomorrow and we can all try again. If this process seems time consuming, imagine the alternative -- an out of control child that others avoid.

Once trust has been built between you and your child, you hope that your child will feel free to ask questions about anything they want to know. If you are comfortable with each other you will be more alert to signs of interest the child shows about his developing body. They may even bring their friends around to talk. Children are drawn to adults who feel comfortable talking with them about growing up. You have a once-in-a-lifetime opportunity to share your priceless gifts of caring and knowledge with the young ones in your life. They will be grateful to you always.

In summary, feeling good about ourselves depends on those who care for us from the beginning of our lives, plus good prenatal care. If we are given closeness, warmth, touching, and our basic needs are met, we learn to reach out to those near us and communicate with them in honest ways. Honest communication builds respect between the child and parents and other caregivers. The child and parents can then listen and talk with each other about many things, including sexuality. Children will listen to the important things they need to know so they can grow into healthy and happy adolescents.

CHAPTER 3

WHY IS IT SO QUIET?

Silence is not necessarily "golden" as the old saying goes. If children are quiet and never ask us questions about sex, for example, we need to ask ourselves, "Why aren't they asking? Children are usually curious about anything grownups know. Sex is no exception. They hear the word spoken at school, on the street and in the media. If children don't get information from parents they are likely to hear it from playmates or as they stand listening to a group of older children whose information is usually incorrect and not what you want your child to be picking up about sex. Even more likely is the chance that your child will see or hear sexual subjects on TV, or from videos or magazines. We cannot screen all of that from their attention. If your child never even hints at wanting you to talk about what that word "sex" means, think about what may be standing in the way. Are you hesitant and uncomfortable with the subject? A child can pick that up very quickly without you having to say a word. Could it be that someone in the family has let the child believe that frank discussion about sexual subjects is a "no-no?" It only takes one time for that "back-off" message to get through to a child all too clearly. So, if you have a child who has never mentioned the "S" word, keep your eyes and ears open and think of ways to approach your child when the time seems right. It's the grownups job to find a time to open up the subject. Your child will be glad that you did.

The "right" time may sneak up on you when you least expect it. Your child may have witnessed a graphic love scene on TV or it may get very quiet in an adjoining room in the house when a cousin or friend comes over to play with your preschooler. Or you may notice two children hidden away in a big box in the day care center playground. When you routinely check to see if they are OK, you may find that they are partly undressed, exploring each other's bodies. This is your moment! The one that can shape their feelings about themselves for years to come and you have no time to think!

21

Some rules of thumb are:

1. Keep your cool. Looks of shock and fright are not useful. The first learning experiences for a child leave the strongest impressions.

2. Remember that the children are behaving normally, doing what children do. They are satisfying their curiosity. Avoid scolding them.

3. Refrain from making negative statements by putting adult labels like "dirty" on the child's exploration.

4. Remember that this exploratory behavior usually lasts only a short time if we're relaxed about it and don't make a big fuss.

5. You can suggest that it is time to join other children in a play activity.

Most children begin to explore their environment and their bodies very early. Even before birth they may suck their thumbs and after birth, touch becomes very important. In the first months, they reach out to touch their parents' faces or a toy, a bright fabric or anything shiny. They are compelled by their developing nervous system to explore all parts of themselves and their surroundings. Sometime or other they will bump into their sexual parts and discover that this part of them feels good to their touch. To the child, every part of their body is good, acceptable and to be valued.

This scenario sounds delightful until an adult labels such behavior as a "no-no," "dirty" or "bad," saying, "Don't touch there. You might hurt yourself"." Since the child feels good about his normal bodily feelings like sucking, being cuddled and stroked, this labeling may produce an unforeseen result. Never label the child's curiosity about genitals as "bad". The child is likely to see him/herself as "bad" and begin to mistrust his/her own feelings or mistrust the adult who is shaming the child. The child's attitude about herself, and later, about sex with her partner, will then be seen as bad or hurtful.

When we understand that curiosity about our bodies is normal, we can be more relaxed about the way we react to a child touching his/her genitals. When babies and toddlers touch themselves, we know that they are following a normal pattern of growth. As children get into the preschool years and language is better developed, they may begin to "play doctor" and compare their bodies with other children. To a child who can understand your words you can say "It does feel good when you touch that part of you, doesn't it? You can let it go at that. Usually, a child is soon ready to go on to some new activity. Their attention span is short.

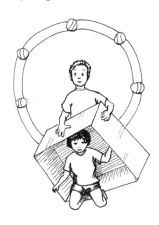

Children's curiosity through the preschool years is greatly lessened if they are able to see what other children's bodies look like. It works well in many homes to let children take baths together, go through the house nude after baths and see their parents nude as they are bathing. Preschools usually have community bathrooms where boys and girls can use the same ones. We need always to be aware not to push these situations on children. If there is embarrassment on the part of the adult or child, it won't work well. As usual, the rule is, follow the lead of the child. We would not want to push children into anything about their bodies that they are uncomfortable with. They can be trusted to do what makes them feel natural and good. If we observe anyone trying to push or force a child into activities that the child resists, that adult must be stopped immediately and the reasons why you are interrupting given calmly. Children let us know by words or by some kind of bodily or facial resistance if they feel pressured. We can teach children to say "no" if they feel pushed to do something they don't like concerning their own bodies.

Teachers, parents and other caregivers will undoubtedly stumble into a time when their child, with a friend or sibling, are exploring each other in a private location indoors or outdoors. You may overhear conversations that let you know that they are playing "doctor" or "house." Once again, stay calm, realizing that if both children are willing participants, this is normal behavior. Depending on the situation you can choose to: (1) let them continue (if they are your children) or (2) say, in a pleasant voice, "It's time to get ready for lunch. Who's hungry?"

If the behavior happens often (and your suggestions don't help) you might talk with the children about the situation, as follows:

ADULT: "What's happening?"
CHILD: "We're playing doctor. We're looking at each other's bottoms".
ADULT: "Is it interesting to see what each other look like?"
CHILD: "Yeah. I've got a penis but she hasn't."

ADULT: "You're right. She's a girl and you're a boy. I have a book about what boys and girls are like. Would you like to help me find it so we can read it?"

You will then, no doubt, have two eager children following at your heels and be able to answer their curiosity by reading the book and discussing it. There are many good books available on this subject. (See Appendix B.) Later on in the day or evening, when you have time to think about it, you can sit down with your child and discuss what happened.

"You and your friend were playing in the box today. What was happening?" The child will give you his version if he feels relaxed and comfortable about it. Then you can say, "I guess you wanted to find out what your friend looked like with no clothes on, right? Did she look different from you? Boys do look different and you may want to know more about that. Let's look at this book that tells about it." It is also important to add, "People don't want to go outside of their house without their clothes on. They want privacy, like when people go to the bathroom. If the child is older, you might ask, "Do you like privacy? It's important to listen to someone when they want privacy. That's called respecting what they want, and people like you better when you respect their privacy."

If children have not learned to be anxious about their sexual organs they will probably not concentrate for any long period on touching that area. They may stimulate themselves occasionally and perhaps want to see what their playmates look like, but then move on to other activities. They are easily distracted. Remember, the more the adult focuses on and shows anxiety about their child's interest in sexuality, the more interesting the whole subject becomes. Once you have answered the child's immediate curiosity they are usually ready to go on to some new activity.

When you react calmly you have shown them that you are not anxious when they show curiosity about their bodies. You have let them know that you are paying attention to their needs and interests; plus you are helping them learn more about the subject. You have not turned a normal behavior into a forbidden activity. If you become aware that a child outside of your family is involved in sex play while under your supervision, try to share what happened with that child's adult caregiver, in a way that will not alarm the adult. Let them know your point of view and that you were in control of the situation. It can be difficult for some parents to understand your approach, but your positive attitude can help and current findings will back you up (Erickson, 1982; Papalia and Olds, 1996.)

Occasionally, children persist in some form of sex play or masturbation every day, over long periods of time. As a teacher of young children, you might notice a child rubbing his/her sex organs during most of a naptime. In that case, there are other factors to consider. You may need to have a parent and their doctor check the child for infection or irritation. The parent may need to get professional advice for any situation beyond what seems like normal behavior. The child may be trying to relieve anxiety and to find comfort through masturbation. If you are the child's teacher or caregiver, hopefully you can find ways to express your concern for the child and suggest that the parent consider why the child is stressed.

The main thing to remember is that children are naturally curious about everything, including their bodies and sexuality. The best thing you can do for them is to treat their curiosity and exploration as a normal activity such as eating, playing or going to the bathroom, while at the same time helping them learn which behaviors are to be kept private. Children have a great capacity for learning what is appropriate in various situations if we explain calmly and lovingly why we are asking for their cooperation. There may be no one else in their lives who will give them that kind of loving guidance as they become adults and enter into a different world. Those children fortunate enough to have such parents are indeed blessed.

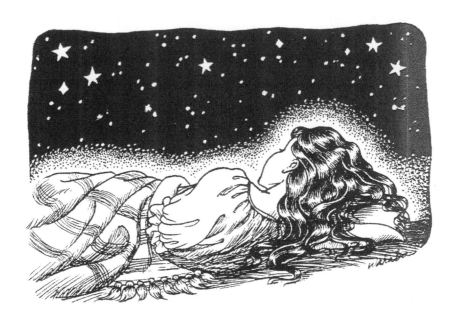

CHAPTER 4

WHERE DID I COME FROM?

Have you ever looked up at the sky on a starry night and wondered how you and your fellow humans got on this earth in the first place? Well, our children's curiosity is just like ours. "Where did I come from?" is a question most parents can expect from their bright-eyed, energetic child in the preschool years. If your first reaction is somewhere between a stare and feeling tongue-tied you are not alone. Take heart. Your child has just passed a growth milestone. If you are asked this question you are lucky to have been given the privilege of helping your child unlock a mystery. Your child asked you, not anyone else, and especially not a casual acquaintance on the street. Now is your chance to have one of those close moments of communication and deepen the trust you both want for each other. It's a moment neither of you may ever forget.

Children ask about where they come from at all different ages. If a new sibling comes along and you actively talk about the baby's prenatal development and preparation for birth, the questions may come at an earlier age: "Well, how did the baby get in there? Can he talk in there and eat? Does he hear me? Did she get in through your belly button?"

It's hard not to laugh or to report to family members in the next room on the cute question your preschooler asked, but do hold back the laughter. Children are really sensitive to what they may see as ridicule, no matter how innocent our intentions. Instead, try a friendly smile and answer your child's question in a straightforward, simple matter. Give just enough information to satisfy your child's curiosity. This is probably not the time to pull out the encyclopedia, or take a sudden trip to the library to check out a stack of books on the subject.

"No, the baby didn't get in through the belly button. See, belly buttons are all closed up, aren't they? The baby began to grow from two very tiny things called an egg and a sperm. When the sperm swam inside the little

27

round egg (you can draw the egg and sperm) the baby looked like this. But right away it started to grow bigger until it began to look like a baby. Remember how Aunt Susan's tummy grew so big when her baby was inside?" At this point, your child may start squirming and be ready to move on to other things. Let the subject rest until the next question comes along.

Somewhere along the way, you may have looked over the available books on birth at bookstores and libraries, or even garage sales. (See suggestions in Appendix B.) Pick books with easy-to-see pictures as well as simple explanations and stories. If you like a book, your child will probably like it as well. If you push too hard on this early education and turn the moment into a tense lecture session, the negative tone will send a clear message to your child: "learning about this stuff is no fun." That's not your aim, of course, but because parents want their child to absorb as much learning as possible, we sometimes push, thereby spoiling the moment that started out as fun and relaxed. Sadly, grown-ups tell us that the pushing by parents and teachers turned them off to books at an early age.

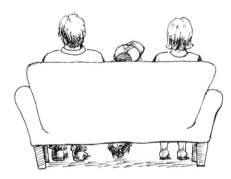

An important fact to remember: Children, like all of us, learn best if they are ready and eager to learn and are relaxed. The moment we pressure a child to sit and "learn" when they are not willing, we are working against the child's natural curiosity. It is just the way our brains are made. The old grim way of drilling facts into the child's head, accompanied by a few yells or a hit on the knuckles when the child "acted up," is as outdated as the dinosaurs. New brain research on learning teaches us a very different way to help children learn. Children learn best when their learning environment is a positive one (Hendrick, 1990).

Success as human being means that we first must feel that we are good and capable. That's another way to describe having good self-esteem, that deep down feeling that we are loveable and we know it. We get that feeling of good self-esteem from our first and ongoing encounters with our parents and others close to us. If we know we are good, others will know it and treat us as loveable. When we are frightened by threats, yelled at and abused in other unspeakable ways, we only learn how to protect ourselves, or get angry, avoid the punisher or get even in all sorts of unacceptable ways. This is why teachers and parents understand that they must give children lots of positive reinforcement, i.e., encouragement and praise, when they are trying to learn something important such as practicing a new skill. For instance:

"I (remember to use **'I'** messages) liked the way you put that puzzle together," or

"You've painted with such bright colors!" or

"You helped me turn the pages of the book while I was feeding your baby sister."

Just noticing the child's efforts is often enough. What the child learned from that book will stay with her longer because the time spent with you was relaxed and satisfying.

When answering your child's question, "Where did I come from?" try to keep your sentences short and simple to match the level of your child's understanding. Remember, too, the child will not be embarrassed unless you are. To a child, learning about sex and reproduction is no different from learning how to put a puzzle together.

The child who was satisfied with the story of the belly button and the sperm at one stage of his understanding will come back eventually with the ultimate question, "But how did the sperm get inside the Mommy?" When you know the child is ready to understand the more complicated details, be sure you are ready to share them without awkwardness or obvious embarrassment. If this is really difficult for you (and it is for many of us), you can rely on those good books you have found at the library or bookstore. Librarians and clerks are very helpful if you get lost in all the titles.

Maybe along with a good children's book, you'd like to have some art materials near by, so you and your child can draw pictures about what he is learning. If your child has seen family members with their clothes off after a bath, perhaps that will make it easier to explain physical differences. You might say:

"Men and boys have penises and women and girls have vaginas. When men and women love each other and feel like being really close, like your Dad and Mom, they want to put their bodies against each other. They may have decided that they are ready to start a new baby together. Maybe they're in bed where it's comfortable. The man's penis gets hard and longer when it rubs against the woman. The closest they can get is for the man to put his penis inside the woman's vagina and, after a lot of wiggling around the penis puts a gooey liquid in the vagina. The liquid has lots of sperm that swim around looking for the woman's egg. Sperm can swim by swishing their tails."

Drawing pictures as you tell this story could help as well as looking at the book. The child could also draw along with you.

"All sperm race to find the egg. The first one that finds the egg goes inside it and a baby starts to grow from that egg with the sperm in it. Once the first sperm gets into the egg, no other sperm can come in and a baby starts to grow."

Some children will be ready to run off and play after the above story is told. Others will want to ask more questions. Children learn and remember things in different ways. (Gardner, 1993). Your child might like to see you draw a picture of the sperm and egg and listen to you as you do most of the talking. Or your child might want to ask lots of questions. Encouraging a child to make a three-dimensional model of the sperm out of clay or play dough might appeal to some children. Don't be surprised if you overhear your child composing a song or poem about eggs and sperm. Children take in and process information, then share it back in their own unique and delightful ways.

There are also children who are more literal in the way they like to learn. If you have a boy who has never seen a vagina, he is likely to ask to see one. or vice versa with a girl. This takes a little tact on your part to help the child realize that people don't like to show children their private parts. You might say, "When women and men love each other, they share those parts of themselves just with each other."

Try to have some pictures or dolls that are anatomically correct to bring out about this time. Or, if you are lucky, you can mention a baby that your child has watched at diaper-changing time. You can assure your child that babies are OK with us watching while their diapers are changed. But, "as children get older," you can point out, "they want more privacy."

If your young children are observing one another as they run around naked after a bath or on a hot day, this is a natural way for them to satisfy their curiosity. It's important to tell them, without causing alarm, that "Each of us is the boss of our own body and we decide when we want to be touched. You can say 'no!' if you don't want to be touched." This applies to kids hitting each other or causing bodily harm in other ways as well. Children don't automatically know their rights or how to communicate their feelings unless we give them some words to use.

As children move along in their development their questions should get more complicated about how the baby grows inside and what it looks like. Use books to help you answer these questions. This is also a good opportunity to talk about the baby's and the mother's need for good food, vitamins, clean air and water and a healthy Mom and Dad so the baby will also grow up to be healthy. You can discuss how all kinds of substance abuse can affect a father's and mother's sperm and egg and cause damage unless they do healthy things. It's important not to frighten your child. Share this information with well chosen words when a child is old enough to understand (Berk, 2002; Allen *et al.*, 1991).

So we see that along with discussions on sex and reproduction, we can begin to talk to our children about nutrition, drug and alcohol abuse and, in general, growing up to be responsible people. You can bring up the fact that you serve nutritious food to the family and ask guests to smoke outside.

It helps to find several ways to illustrate the information you are sharing with your child and to tie that information into something they already understand. Reminding them of something they did or learned earlier is a good way for them to remember as you add new information on that same subject. Also anytime children can make a model, draw a picture or in any way practice something they are learning, the better their chance of remembering the new learning:

- **I hear it and I listen.**
- **I see it and I remember.**
- **I do it and I understand.**

If a child surprises you by saying, "Hey, let's do it," after hearing your explanation about the egg and sperm, you can say, "No, that's something adults do when they find someone to love and want to have babies with. When you're older it will be easier to understand." Of course, you will be having lots of future conversations as they grow older.

Remember that the beautiful part of discussing sex and reproduction with your children at an early age is that **they** are not embarrassed by it. That makes it easier for you. After your first talks together, it will be natural and normal to discuss these subjects. Teens today say that the ability to talk openly with their parents is one of the most important factors in helping them get through the

31

teen years without an unwanted pregnancy or other problems like sexually transmitted diseases. They say they feel safer and more confident about growing up. Current research backs up what these teens have said (Kaiser Foundation Survey, 1996). The more quality sex information teens get, the more responsibly they behave and the less chance they have of getting pregnant. The old idea that the more they know, the more sexually active they will be, is just not accurate. Our children look to us for leadership and values and they are better able to set goals and be responsible and be in control of their own life if we are close to them and share our feelings and information with them. Robert Gunn, M.D. (1996) Department of Health Services in San Diego, says that "teens want their parents to initiate discussions about (sex) and parental advice is taken seriously."

Also remember that you do not have to do all this educating alone. Include other members of the family. Let them know about your plans for discussing sex and reproduction with your child. You can have family time as you talk and look at books and watch TV shows explaining these topics. The research is showing that TV doesn't have to have a destructive influence on children. If parents know what the child is watching, they can comment about topics that puzzle children (Comstock and Paik, 1991). A child can learn to understand and be critically aware of material that deals with, for example, selling useless products, or promoting pollution, violence and sex. These subjects are available as an everyday diet for even young children whose parents use TV as a baby sitter. The young child's brain is absorbing all of this at a fast pace and their values are being shaped by everything in their environment (White House Conference, 1997).

Parents are speaking out more and more to their PTA's, their lawmakers and to the press about their concerns over violence on TV. Children learn from the parents as they watch them write letters or call the White House or Congress to tell them their views. Children who see this kind of modeling by their parents will be more likely to take part in the democratic process in our local, state and national governments when they are grown. This way, they can be a powerful influence on their communities.

Remember to include grandparents in your child's education as well, and any other extended family members who want to help. They may jump right in and add to the family discussions. If not, at least they will be able to observe and share their opinions, we hope, in a helpful manner. If not, it's probably better to be sure they are not in the room. If grandparents are truly supportive, as the children get older they might talk to their grandparent or other relative, when

32

they don't always feel comfortable talking to their parents. Margaret Mead, the great anthropologist said, "Children need a close relative so they can run away from home around the block" (Mead, 1974).

It's a compliment to the parent when they see their children also asking for assistance from other extended family members. When grown children move out into the adult world we hope that they will feel comfortable asking for, and accepting help from those outside the immediate family. We know that this kind of help could be extremely useful to them.

However, when children get information or advice from others outside the home we may find that they come home with information that is harmful and full of errors. This is why daily conversations with your child are so important. "How was your day?" discussions are a great way to keep you alert to what is going on in your child's life. Good listening without harsh judgments will keep your child talking (See Chapter 1 on Communication) and will help you recognize danger signals and confusion in your child's mind. Good listening doesn't mean you necessarily approve, but at least you will know what's happening. Recently an adult told his friends that he used to come home with all kinds of hair-raising stories about what he and his teenage friends did for fun. His parent was smart enough to listen, raise an eyebrow at times and then keep listening so appropriate action or advice could be given at the right moment. As a result, this man and his parent remain close throughout their lives.

Of course, parents have the responsibility of seeing that their children are getting the best and most accurate information available for their age level. Schools need to be careful to explain to parents about any sex education that is being offered in schools and parents have the right to review the material and sign an approval slip. Much of it is very useful and helpful to young teens. However, teenagers continue to ask for more "real-life" information about the emotional side of sexuality. They want to know how they can deal with pressure and feelings of loneliness and rejection. They may fear rejection if they say "no" to sexual activity with their girlfriend or boyfriend. The next chapters will explore these problems in depth. Parents, remember that you are the person your child would most like to talk to and learn from. The responsibility sometimes seems overwhelming, but the lifelong communication bond you build with your child now is irreplaceable.

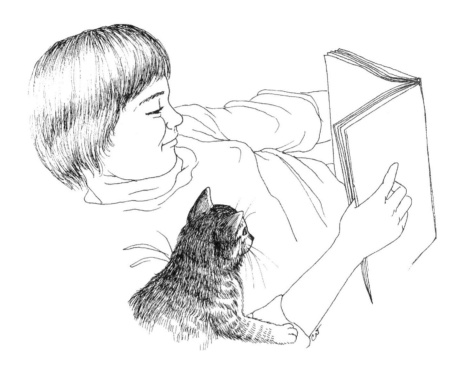

CHAPTER 5

WHY DO I FEEL DIFFERENT TODAY?

As parents, we probably breathe a sigh of relief when we see our children dressing themselves, going to school and taking on increasing responsibilities around the house. We know that they are learning how to navigate in the world without our always having to peek over their shoulder. We might find that we now have a little time for ourselves as well. But keep in mind, whatever stage our child is now in, another stage is on its way. We are all too aware that after the child's middle years, adolescence is that next stage.

The word "adolescence" used to strike terror into parents' hearts. We are now seeing evidence of teens actually having fun and rewarding times with their parents. Why? Because, it seems, their parents have uncovered some secrets of communication that work with teens. It's not surprising that parents who have the most success in enjoying their teenagers, began good family communications early.

If you were able to start off your relationship with your child as described in the first chapter of this book, you already have some good things going for you:

1.   You are friends as well as the primary guide for your child.
2.   You and your child like to be together.
3.   You respect and understand your child's needs and can listen to and care about those needs.
4.   You know that each of your children is a different individual and those differences have to be taken into account if you want to hear your child's needs and be heard by your child.

But if, for whatever reason, you and your young teen are not comfortable talking about certain subjects, don't be discouraged. When as parents we truthfully share our doubts and uncertainties with our children, they are most likely ready to listen and help us through our own awkwardness. They are usually very good at forgiving.

35

Parents sometimes say, "But my child won't tell me what he feels." Children often don't have words to say how they feel so they can't answer directly. Your job may be to interpret what the child would like to say but can only show you, in subtle ways. Watch for clues. When our babies were hungry they didn't have to say, "Pass the milk, please," for us to get the idea. The same applies with older children. We can tell when our child is happy. His body and face are relaxed or smiling. His eyes sparkle, he may give hugs, and he usually has some new idea he wants to try out again! That's "happy." We also can see when a frown, a tense jaw, or frightened eyes cloud our child's facial expressions. They cry or they give us the silent treatment, and we can almost see that dark thunder cloud hovering overhead.

Sometimes, however, unless we're watching closely, we may miss the clues. Sadly, an opportunity for real communication passes us by. The child, unaware that parents can't read minds, may go away convinced that his parent doesn't listen. Yet we may not have noticed that troubled feelings were building within our child. Later, we can let the child know that we didn't ignore her feelings on purpose and that it helps us when the child lets us know how she feels and how we can help.

When that change called "adolescence" begins to happen, and it can start very subtly, your ability to read your child's facial and body language really pays off. Let your child know what you think you're seeing. (A guess is usually the safe way to go.) "Does that frown mean you aren't happy about doing your chores now?" or at another time, "Your eyes look sad to me. Want to talk about anything?"

If this way of approaching your child is new to you, don't be discouraged if you get some funny looks the first time you try it. Just keep at it, until your teenager is convinced you are serious. The beauty of this way of communicating is that you don't have to solve all your child's problems. Many times pre-adolescents just need an older, wiser person to come to with their feelings and ideas. Grandparents can be great for this. Your teenager will let you know when they want advice and when they **don't** want it. Watch for those subtle clues, like an impatient look or a turn away from you. They may not say it in words, but the feelings are clear if we are observant.

Parents know that keeping quiet is a difficult task. After all, we had to be ready to offer positive words when our child learned to walk. We probably had to yell when they were about to step into the street. If health and safety is involved we will always speak out. Otherwise, it is helpful to think before we speak unless our advice has been requested.

As young teens mature, they depend on their parents to show them, by modeling and setting limits, how to take on more responsibilities. Your friendship with them also matures. For instance, we can understand why it's important to listen to a good friend without giving unwelcome advice. So it is with our budding adolescents. However, no parent we know is willing to clam up completely and nod constantly as their young adolescent pours out their problems.

Parents should feel free to voice their opinions. Just be sure the word "opinion" is stressed. Beginning a sentence with, "I believe, I hope, I wish," etc. can be useful. Opinions filter through a child's brain more easily and with less resistance than a parental order. They want to be in control of their decisions and will take our opinions strongly into consideration if we offer them in a calm, caring way. If the subject at hand concerns health and safety, of course parents give more than opinions. They give reasons and consequences growing out of their own teen experience and their knowledge. They are not afraid to set limits and consistently stick by them. We know that teens may break our rules, but we at least have taken a firm stand, shared our values and cared enough to make and enforce rules for our children. At some point, they are likely to remember those values and use them without our always knowing about it. When our children do make mistakes, they need to know they can depend on us to back them up and help them do better next time. "A parent cannot lose when they make mistakes. The only way a parent can lose is to give up" (Intermountain Health Care, 1993).

Let's assume that good communication is taking place between you and your young teen. You notice subtle or not so subtle changes in your child's body and behavior. Research shows that some girls are beginning puberty at 8 years of age. The average age for girls to begin menstruation is 12 and for boys the onset of puberty is on the average, at 14 years of age (Malina and Bouchard, 1991; Tanner, 1990).

These changes take many parents by surprise. They know it's coming but -- so soon? They may have trouble accepting the fact that their sweet little baby will soon be grown and most likely, gone from home. It's a big adjustment. The thought of going through this adolescent phase with their child may stir up old hurtful memories of the parents' own teenage years. Some parents try to ignore these signs of change in their budding teen and are caught up later in a crisis with a teenager in trouble. Teenagers want us to recognize that they are no longer our little children, but still are our children. Remember, that we have to read their facial and body language. Make it easier on yourself by expecting and welcoming adolescence with a sense of humor. You'll feel more in control and so will your child.

Expecting and welcoming adolescence still won't give you all the answers but at least you'll be mentally alert -- a little like a baseball player waiting in the outfield for a ball to come her way, prepared to move in any direction.

If open communication is the rule in your house, your children may tell you when they feel strange or different or as they begin to see changes in their body. If you've already talked about all this and read books together, they will probably be excited to see that it is really happening to them. It's very important that we appreciate their excitement and interest in themselves without teasing and poking fun. Young teenagers often take themselves very seriously and most haven't developed much of a sense of humor about themselves. Hormonal changes cause feelings to be supersensitive. Can you remember when you went through adolescence? And those of us who are older, remember menopause? During these

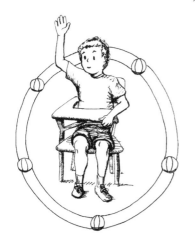

changes we can't tolerate too much outside pressure. So tread somewhat softly on your teen's tender feelings. They will thank you, perhaps silently, for it.

One of the best attitudes you could have as you observe your teenager's hormonal flip-flop is one of celebration and pride that he or she is doing what all humans do, growing up. This is not to suggest that when your child is moaning and groaning over a voice change or budding breasts (when no other girl in the sixth grade has any) you dismiss it as "only a phase." But, in general, keeping an upbeat, optimistic attitude can be a good thing. Most children like to hear stories of when their parents suffered through their teen years. Try some of those and see if they are welcomed. If you see rolling eyes and a look that says "Oh, no, not again!" then maybe stories are not the way to go. Keep your eye on the teen!

If the atmosphere around your house is upbeat concerning normal teenage development, chances are that your teen will join in with the same attitude. There will still be good days and bad days. You may find your daughter dressing in high-heels, hose and lipstick one day, while cuddling in bed with her teddy bear the next or wanting to sit in your lap (even when they are approaching six feet in height). One 12-year old we know decided to take a baby bottle to junior high school and started a new fad among her friends. Wisely, that parent bit her lip, stayed silent and the fad died out within two weeks.

It's hard to view our children as children when they look so big and often try to fool us with deadpan expressions or words of wisdom which we may mistakenly think they are following. Not necessarily so. Remember back in the toilet training days? We thought that when they stayed dry for four nights in a row, we were home free. We joyfully put on their training pants then found the bed soaking wet the next morning. It seems that development happens in small steps, some of them backwards, before moving ahead.

A special area of concern for adolescents is their need for acceptance by their peers. You'll know this is happening when most of their free time is spent on the phone or "hanging out" with their buddies almost anywhere and anytime they can manage it. That's when family outings become their second choice, unless a friend can go along. A lot of time is spent in front of the mirror while their hair and clothing choices are not what we parents had in mind when we dreamed about our children becoming adults. Expect your adolescent to try to look, act and think differently than you expect. Try to understand that they have to see your ways as "old-fashioned" while they question your every opinion. A parent could be the Angel Gabriel and still be unable to satisfy their teenager. It's nature's way of assuring that teenagers will grow into their own persons and establish a life as individuals separate from their parents. There are exceptions to this scenario. Some children pass through this separation phase less stressfully than do others.

Another way to ease the stress for you and your teens is by inviting their friends to come to **your** house. If a teen can invite friends home and the parents welcome them, these friends will most likely accept the invitation, especially if they are given some space. It can be scary out on the streets for teens. If there are no after-school programs available and there is someone at your house you trust to supervise, your home can be a safe haven for teens. Statistics show that the highest crime rate for teens occurs between 3 and 6 in the afternoon. What better way to know your teens' friends than to invite them to enjoy backyard picnics, (with **their** choice in music), and games, while munching on cookies? The trick is to be there but not to be too visible so they can feel free to be themselves, knowing you will protect them if trouble arises. They can be advised ahead of time that no alcohol is to be served or other drugs tolerated and that you will be around to help if needed. This open door policy, (within limits, of course) may seem like an invasion of your privacy. But peace of mind may be your reward if you announce and back up your limits firmly (hopefully, while smiling). You then have a better chance of knowing where your child is and who his friends are down the block.

Since we are not cats, dogs or bees who say goodbye to their young quickly, we have to find ways to live through this long human growing up process. If you can keep your sense of humor when it seems your teenager: (1) would rather be anywhere with his friends than at home; (2) lets you know, less than tactfully, that you are out of step with the times; (3) tests at least once, just about every rule you have firmly set down -- then you will probably be accepted as a "cool" parent. Hold the line and enforce rules consistently. Keep the lines of communication open. Chances are, your teenager will trust and respect you and will come to you with questions about his body changes and sexuality.

An open line of communication sounds like a great idea, but it can also cause worry and anguish for some parents. Parents who fear talking or knowing what their teens are doing probably never had an open relationship with their own parents. These parents may rarely or never make time to talk or listen, especially in sensitive areas like sexuality. Maybe they hope it will go away, or that someone else (like the school) will step in to help. Teenagers tell us that that's how they got into trouble sexually. They want love and limits, yes, but they also want information. Without facts and feelings from parents, children wade into a murky world of sexually transmitted diseases, teen pregnancy, drugs and crime. No one deserves such burdens, especially our youth who are so new to life. The answers are out there and adults have the responsibility of showing them where those answers can be found, even if we feel awkward and strange at first. Remember, our children have a great way of putting us at ease if we take the first difficult steps and open up the subject.

Ideally, young teens have already talked with parents and seen books from the library or at school on male and female body characteristics. If they don't know, it's time to discuss it, along with the moral and practical responsibilities toward themselves and others. Being grown-up and parenting a child is a huge

40

responsibility. Insight about sexual relationships doesn't come naturally to a child. We have to talk about it and give the child a chance to do some hands-on activities in preparation. Sadly, too many parents and school personnel think they have done their part when they cover the nuts and bolts and "plumbing" lectures on sex. Most children already learned that from books or friends. What they don't know is how to respond when they are pressured to have sex or think it might be fun to have a sweet little baby to care for. When these feelings are never discussed, the young person may think that they are the only one with such a feeling or that there is no way out. They have little experience in knowing that, with patience, problems can be worked out.

THE "M" WORD

Sooner or later you are going to have to deal with the subject of masturbation. Either you will be asked a question about it or you will discover that your child or grandchild has been experimenting just like most other children. Consider yourself lucky and trusted if your youngster confides in you by asking questions about masturbation. Even if your child or adolescent uses a slang word such as "jerking off," rather than the clinical term we are using here, it's best to avoid all appearance of embarrassment or shame in discussing the subject.

We realize that our generation, and even our children's generation, may not feel comfortable with this subject. However, if you are seriously interested in helping your child grow up with a healthy sense of sexuality, you need to be prepared to discuss masturbation with the same open attitude without guilt or shame that you show for all the other areas of sexuality you discuss with your youngster.

First of all, let's be realistic in recognizing that in today's America, almost every boy and many girls will discover masturbation long before they mature into adults. As a matter of fact, various studies indicate that more than 80% of boys have masturbated to orgasm by age fifteen. Though the rates among girls are much lower, there is some evidence to suggest that at least one out of five girls has also discovered masturbation by age fifteen (Kinsey *et al.*, 1953). It has also been found that girls generally add masturbation to their sexual behavior after they have begun sexual intercourse with a partner. As both males and females mature, they expand in their variety of sexual outlets, including masturbation. For example, unlike the impression most people seem to have that masturbation is for "losers," well-documented research shows that masturbation is more frequent among those who have the greatest number of other, and very legitimate, sexual outlets. It is reported that

41

"nearly 85% of men and 45% of women who were living with a sexual partner said they had masturbated in the past year" (Michael *et al.*, 1994).

It is clear that the recognition that human beings enjoy masturbation has come full circle from the almost universal disapproval of the 19th century when John Harvey Kellogg (the inventor of cornflakes), and other prominent Victorians advocated drastic measures, including male circumcision, physical restraints for boys, and even cliterodectomies, the most cruel sexual mutilation for girls caught in the act or suspected of masturbation.

Most sex therapists, psychiatrists and psychologists now agree that masturbation is every bit as legitimate as other "normal" sexual activities. Teenagers report that they feel safer using these mutual techniques to pleasure their partners to avoid unwanted pregnancies especially when they don't feel ready. They can learn about their sexuality in non-threatening ways without pressure to have intercourse before they feel comfortable, which often means within a committed relationship and marriage.

Another crucial element in learning about sexuality is the way our children develop their attitudes toward sexuality in general, and toward self-pleasuring in particular. Most people still have feelings of embarrassment, shame, or guilt about most, if not all, sexual activities. Gagnon and Simon in their book *SEXUAL CONDUCT* (1973) state "that learning about sex in our society is learning about guilt." So, then, learning to manage sexuality helps us "learn how to manage guilt."

This means that we, as adult caregivers, play a very important role in helping youngsters avoid the kinds of guilt feelings and shame so many of us have experienced, interfering with the sort of healthy attitudes about sexuality we would like to encourage. We obviously do not want to pass on some of the sexual "hang-ups" and disabilities we inherited from earlier generations. Being honest with our children really is a much better way.

A teenager's overriding, most powerful need is to be loved, cherished and held close as they go through their powerful bodily changes. If they do not receive that closeness and information from wise grownups, they will always go for the closeness wherever they can find it, with or without the safeguards they need. The chapters ahead suggest ways to talk with your young teenager about these challenges so you can better prepare them to cope with all the choices and feelings ahead.

CHAPTER 6

TALK TO YOUR YOUNG TEEN -- START NOW

"Teens who are close to their parents are more likely to remain sexually abstinent, postpone intercourse and have fewer partners and to use contraceptives."
Miller et al., 1998

We want to help our children understand about sex and we want to protect them from harm. Parents and young teens are subjected to more information on the subject of sex today than at any time in human history. Teens have many more choices and the freedom to make them than did their parents. Some of these choices involve threats to our children's health and their future well-being. Even though there are effective ways to steer our children around them, scary realities like sexually transmitted diseases and unwanted pregnancies affect far too many of our teenagers.

For many parents, the communication gap seems to widen with the sudden arrival of adolescence. We may not be prepared for this communication problem. The sweet little kid we played with and protected suddenly has developed an independent streak and does not seem to mind telling us so. Adolescents soon let us know how irritated they are with our "inadequacies." Remember the first time that forceful "no" came out of the mouth of your two-year old? You may have thought it was cute then, knowing it was a stage that hopefully would be outgrown. It is hard to do, but try to see your adolescent's criticisms like that, too. They **have** to see us as separate from them and to point out our mistakes in their eyes, so that their own identity can blossom. They are then able to make a healthy separation, and if we are supportive of their new self-image, family life runs more smoothly. Adolescents who are allowed a reasonable space to verbally express themselves, are more likely to come back to a stronger respect for the traditional values of their families. Teens who are met with angry disapproval may get "stuck" with dangerous rebellion and lifetime distancing from their parents.

43

PARENTS, YOUR TEENS ARE WATCHING

The critical attitudes and behavior teens may demonstrate to their parents are only a small part of what is really going on under the surface. They watch us closely when we least expect it and notice just about **everything** we do. Not that they will share that fact with us. They are compelled by Mother Nature to grow up and to be their own persons. Yet we are their closest role models and best allies. We hope they will like what they see about us. Take comfort in knowing that your teen's annoying habits are not the finished product, and that he or she is "in process." It may make it easier to accept your teen at that moment. We are hoping for signs of maturity later on, of course. Time and patience are needed during this period with the realization that this phase will not last forever.

STEER CLEAR OF SUBTLE BEHAVIORAL AGGRESSION

Child guidance professionals, many of whom may also be parents, tell us that children do better when they are accepted for who they are, while at the same time are given consistent limits so that they can live more harmoniously with others. Scolding, nagging, labeling or humiliating behavior toward a child simply causes that child to retreat. One psychologist has named these kinds of negative actions as behavioral aggression. We use these negative methods thinking that they will help our children behave better (Hackbert, 2000). Hackbert maintains that the behavior we give attention to will continue to occur in the future. However, the more we as parents continue those negative behaviors the more the children will retreat, clam up, and steer clear of our company so that we have less influence in their lives. If we want them to consider our point of view, we need to swallow our annoyance and try active listening (See Chapter 1). Sometimes our children just need us to be there, listening to them without giving advice, as a good friend might do. Of course, as their parents we are there to state and enforce our rules and limits with love. If we continuously build good will with our teens, we can earn their respect. When we firmly state and enforce the rules with love, our teens will most likely be willing to cooperate. Children of all ages want firm, fair limits and our approval. Sometimes they use our rules to their advantage with their friends. As parents of teenagers, we remember times when our children felt good about telling a visiting friend to "say goodnight because our parents said the party was over." Quite often, they were the ones who really wanted the friends to go.

TEENS WANT TO LEARN FROM YOU FIRST!

Perhaps you have steered successfully through the rough waters of basic communication with your explosive or perhaps even sullen teen. Look for an opportunity to talk with her or him about personal and emotional areas like sex. Chances are this is harder for you to discuss than any other subject. We remember the awkwardness we felt with our parents when they approached the same subject with us. The "S" word was a forbidden topic for many and we still find ourselves stumbling about for the best words to use.

Any poll taken these days tells us that teens prefer learning about sex from their parents but they also don't expect that this will happen in their family. In a 1996 poll done by the Kaiser Foundation, most teens stated that they knew how girls got pregnant but they wanted to know about feelings and values surrounding sex and they wished they could talk to their parents about it and if not their parents, then their teachers. Typically, teens turn to their mothers to discuss sex. Fathers have traditionally not taken the lead in this area, but children need to know how both parents feel. Anytime that feels right is a good time to talk. In addition, there is no one "right way" to discuss such an important subject. Just try to use language your child can understand.

Some parents express the fear that if they bring up the subject of sex, they may be putting ideas of promiscuity into their young teens' heads. Studies done in recent years say that this just is not true. The best kind of sex education tends to delay teenager's early sex experiences, not hasten it.

We know also that teenagers already have plenty of ideas in their heads unless they have been living on a desert island. They also have lots of questions, fears and anxieties about sex. Not only are their bodies pushing them in that direction, they are also surrounded by many kinds of contradictory messages about sex coming from the media.

It would be surprising if teens weren't confused. They are hearing information that says, "Don't have sex, but if you do, be careful." We, as parents, owe our children the honesty and respect of giving them straight and real answers. This is not "glamorizing sex" as some might fear. Physician Drew Pinsky says, "We are confronting behavior. The idea is to climb into our teen's culture and feel what they feel" (Barovick, 1998). Otherwise, how can we talk with them and understand their point of view, the first step in solving a problem.

The evidence is in that early sex education reduces early sexual experimentation and teen pregnancy. In sections of the United States where comprehensive sex education exists, teenage pregnancy and diseases have declined (Santelli, 1998). It is important to note that wherever these rates have gone down, adults say that they have made sure their young people have had plenty of interesting activities to hold their interest, and attentive grown ups to be involved. Then the temptation to fill the time with sex, drugs, and problem behaviors is greatly reduced.

Our children want and need time with us and it is our job to plan time with them, if we want the bond we have built together to stay strong. Hopefully, you are succeeding in building a bond of trust with your young teenager. It takes all your patience and lots of "walking in their moccasins." Hang in there. The future rewards will be great.

MEDIA HYPE CAN BE SCARY

Parents who read and hear about teenage rates of delinquency and pregnancy can get jittery about their own child's future. Even though the media tend to exaggerate and sensationalize stories about troubled teens in order to sell their products, only a few teens make the headlines in this way. Those teens who get in trouble are crying out for adult guidance and attention. It is up to us adults to find a way to relieve their pain or else real tragedies will continue to occur. No teen really enjoys delinquent behavior. In the early stages, teens typically try for attention in less dramatic ways. Later, if their needs are ignored, they may go on to more extreme behavior, even including assault and murder on school grounds. How tragic that those children may be driven to depression, suicide and murder before they get the kind of attention they need. We must learn to notice the warning signs well before desperation causes them to try extreme behavior.

Watch for behaviors that psychologist Charles Hannaford (1987) and other health professionals have identified as serious:

1.   "Rebellious behavior or withdrawal behaviors."
2.   "Changes in clothing and music which copy the drug culture."
3.   "Lack of successful school performance."
4.   "Quick to anger and refusal to talk about friends or to share their activities with the family."

TEENS TRY TO COPE

Tom McMahon, a father of two and a professor of counseling, has written a book, *TEEN TIPS, A PRACTICAL SURVIVAL GUIDE FOR PARENTS WITH KIDS 11 THROUGH 19*. He asked parents of happy, healthy teens

46

across the country to share their tips on coping. Among his most important findings was that 75% of these teens have healthy images of themselves. Dr. McMahon says, "The more I learn about adolescents, the more I marvel at how well they cope."

Perhaps they cope as well as they do because they watch the adults around them and try to seek out good role models. Our children are watching us all and we hope we can be a good example for them. Children imitate what they see in the adult world including their attitudes about sex. The problem is they may know the mechanics of sex but they are usually not mature enough to understand the feelings and responsibilities that go along with sexual behavior. Their sexual drives are leading them but the caution signs are not yet in place. That's where parents and teachers play such an important part. Their influence with teens is very strong **if** they can talk openly together.

Junior High counselors report that, in their experience, young teens seem almost nonchalant about sex as if it is no big deal, unlike their elders who become nervous as soon as the "S" word is mentioned. Perhaps these teens are attempting to look "cool" and in control. Look more deeply and we may see a frightened, uncertain child.

Young teens may think they are really sophisticated about sex. But they have very little experience in how to talk about their feelings with their peers if, for instance, they feel pushed into becoming sexual with peers before they are ready. How can they still be popular and remain abstinent?

These are hard questions to deal with, but if we do not ask them early on, our children may stumble blindly into all kinds of problems while getting their information from confused peers or from street "wisdom." Teens may put a lot of effort into trying to look and act grown-up. They're just practicing their new adult roles, so don't be fooled. Underneath they are often 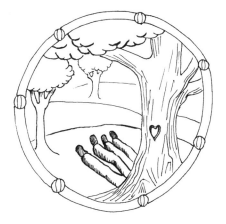 confused and scared at the newness of it all. They will be very relieved to have a parent bring up the subject even if they act somewhat disgusted with you at the time.

Robert Gunn (1996) suggests we look for the "teachable moments" when we know we have our young teen's attention and interest. Seize the moments when they are listening, not heading for the front door. If they ask questions, that's even better. We need to make sure we take them seriously and take the time to answer their questions. And it is perfectly all right to answer with a straightforward, "I don't know" if necessary. That's an honest answer and teens will appreciate it. Good reference books that answer your questions can help (see Appendix A).

Remember that your child likes to hear stories about your own experiences. The important point to keep in mind is to keep the lines of communication open. By being able to converse about the subject of sex, you send the message that it is not a forbidden subject and that you care about your child's feelings. A good way to begin a conversation with your child is to use the "I feel" approach. They listen when you say, "I believe" or "I am concerned that" or " it really bothers me" when discussing your concerns about your child's behavior. Teens listen to feelings, not lectures.

Try to avoid negative phrases like, "Don't come in late" or "Don't have sex" which almost programs them to try it. It spotlights the "forbidden" activity even more. A more positive and effective way to say the same thing might be, "Curfew is at 11. See you then," or "I believe teens need to take steps to have responsible sex," or "I believe it is a good idea for people to wait to have sex until they are ready to decide together what kind of a future they want to build." It helps if a family member or a friend's experience can be used as a good example. You may find yourself in a one-way conversation with a teen who won't respond verbally. Be pleasant, speak your truth, and then move on -- the teenager has heard you.

Young adults who take our classes let us know every semester how much they wished that their parents could have been straightforward with them about sex. Margaret Mead (1974) pointed out in one of her lectures that she believed that sex should be discussed at the dinner table just like any other subject. That attitude may seem extreme to some, but the idea is to take the awkwardness out of dealing with sex in our parent-teen talks.

When we asked our 16-year-old granddaughter to give us some tips on how teens liked to be informed about sex by their parents, the answers at the top of her list were the following:

1. Avoid lecturing, instead you may want to tell stories about your own early teen experiences and feelings, and "how I felt at that age." As

adults, we need to take time for them. Our time could not be used more wisely.

2. When our granddaughter was asked how adults might begin a talk concerning sexuality with a teen, she suggested, "Let your teen know your feelings and beliefs about being sexual even if you don't think they will agree. They want and need to know your feelings and why you feel that way." We as adults know that honesty is the best and most secure way to deal with our children. When we are clear about our beliefs and values about sexual conduct, our teens will have a much easier time developing a set of standards for themselves.

When we say, "You may or may not agree with my point of view on this, but I want you to know how I feel and why I feel that way," it is a way of letting teens know that, although they will not be under our supervision at all times, they will know our opinions and values. There is no guarantee they will take our advice. Our most powerful tool is "friendly persuasion" to help them see the logic of actions they might choose. If we lecture and shout they are likely to ignore us and they could end up choosing the opposite behavior just to show that we can't "run their life."

Whatever rules you make, such as age of dating, curfew hours, or chaperoned parties, be clear with your teen and stick to your word if the rules are ignored. Let the penalty fit the violation and spell out the rules beforehand. It is important that your teen does not get the impression that you expect him or her to goof-up. That is an invitation to prove you right and get negative attention from you, which to them may feel better than getting no attention at all. Try also to avoid reminding your teen of their past goof-ups. Nothing can be done to correct those and this can easily seem like a put down.

When the time comes to make rules, sit down in a relaxed, friendly way when there is no time schedule pressuring you, and talk about the problem. It is very important to let your teen talk about concerns and feelings. Listening without interrupting and judging will encourage your teen to be more cooperative and they may then follow your lead and listen to you! Teens need to know that there are rules for the whole family and that there are clear and logical reasons for these rules. The old "do it because I say so" doesn't work anymore, especially if you want your kids to respect you and learn to cooperate. The rules we need to really enforce usually center on the health and safety of all family members and respect for the family's schedule. When your teen comes in after their curfew hour, someone at home is probably losing sleep and stressing out waiting for them.

Consistent rule setting and enforcement is an art that parents can learn. They will then reap the rewards when family members feel they are working together towards harmony at home. When teens challenge your rules, be ready for a variety of creative arguments. Be prepared to repeat yourself many times, always in your steady and friendly voice. A little humor helps like "I know I'm the worst ogre on the block when I insist that you are home by 10:30 PM." Especially be prepared to state clearly the reasons why and the consequences of breaking the rules.

"I hear you when you say the other kids' parents let them stay out later, but I'm **your** parent and I only have responsibility for your safety," or, "I'm sure you would rather have a party without your parents in the house, but we are responsible for what happens in this house. We can be in another part of the house and not interrupt unless you need us." Believe it or not, teens like to know someone is in charge and that their privacy will be respected unless they need a parent to intervene, even though they may act outraged that you are in the house at all. Is it any wonder that some parents are tempted to send their children down the block to hang out with friends? Unfortunately, some parents use that as a quick solution to conflict. However, later on, they may find that the problem has multiplied and requires a lot more energy to solve it. Deal with a problem as soon as you can while solutions are still easy to find.

PARENTS CAN BE TONGUE TIED- WHEN THE SUBJECT IS SEX

In the best of all possible situations, our young teen will come to us with questions about sex and we gladly answer them. However, parents may have to be the ones to bring up the topic. Our teen grandchild suggests the following to help parents through what may be an awkward beginning:

"I need to talk to you about some important matters about sex. I don't exactly know how to do this. Maybe because my parents didn't know how to talk to me about it either. But maybe we can help each other."

Then let your teen respond and accept whatever they offer you. Take it at a slow pace. When we can let teens see that we don't know it all, they can relax a little and feel closer to us because it's a safe guess that they are confused or scared or both. They know their parents are experienced and

50

they would rather hear their own parent's experiences and feelings than anyone else's, especially when the subject of sex is so new to them. Remember, it is not necessary or desirable to tell your teenager the details of your own intimate relationships in order to help them understand about sex. Just as you answered only their immediate questions like "Where did I come from?" when they were small, you can again simplify your answers. "Couples have private times which only they want to share with each other."

These discussions need to start early, because by age 11 and 12 many children have already heard a lot from their friends and the media. Always assume that your child knows more than you think. Chances are they do! Let your child know that you realize he or she may have learned a lot already. Teens like to be given credit for knowing a lot! But what they do not know and understand (unless you tell them) is how this whole area of sexuality is seen from your perspective as an older and more experienced adult.

We want to help them understand about love and affection that grows into long-term relationships where sex is experienced by two people who respect each other and want to have a life together. You could say, after viewing a TV program together, "There was a lot of information about how sex happens between a man and woman but they didn't talk about feelings a couple might have about each other. Would you like to talk about that part with me?" If your child's answer is "yes," be honest about how you believe a love relationship works. Talk about your own in general terms, perhaps. "Your Dad and I got to know each other for a long time. We had fun together and we got to know each other's families. We finally realized we respected each other and liked to be together and to be close." The details will be different for each family. If your child says "Not right now" to such a discussion, let it go with "O.K., if you decide you'd like to talk about it later, let me know." Being too eager to share information can be a turn off-for some teens.

Let your teen know you respect his or her ability to be responsible and make choices, then let him or her know that you recognize that growing up can be tough and confusing. Each person has to make and live with individual personal choices. Every choice we make has a consequence and its good to learn and consciously think about what might happen before we proceed. Talking it over helps us make good choices.

After you have a chance to find out just how much your teen really does know and understand about sex, without pushing too hard and being accused of prying, you might say, "I have faith in you that you will make responsible choices so that you and others won't get hurt and you can be safe and healthy. It's important to know some information about staying healthy and safe, and we can talk about that so you will be able to take care of yourself and the person you care about." Then you can share in a straightforward way what responsible sex is all about and how they can protect themselves, including everything from abstinence to safe-sex precautions and the use of birth control according to your particular values. The next chapter gives suggestions for ways to explain these essential topics.

It is so very important to let your child know as soon as you feel they can really understand, that intimate relationships are different from affection shown a friend. When your children were very young you helped them respect and care for their bodies. Your family members and friends show affection and respect for each other in ways the growing child can see, such as hugging, kissing, pats on the back, giving neck rubs, etc. We want a child to grow up knowing the difference between a handshake and holding hands. One is a show of respect; the other is a show of affection. Intimate sexual relations, we hope they can understand, are much deeper than just the sexual act. If a couple gets to know each other well and shows love and respect, then sex is much more satisfying and enjoyable. We want our children to know that the sex by itself, without affection and respect for their partner, is a less satisfying experience. Unless two people have that close feeling and respect, the relationship they create together may not be as close and respectful either. Even though we may wonder if our children can understand, it is important that they hear it from us more than once.

The sad fact is, if families cannot show affection for one other, then the children will search for that affection outside the home as they get to be teens. They may think that what they see on TV or the movies is what sex is all about. Teens seeking outside affection will look for anyone who offers them attention. These often turn out to be adults or young adults pressuring younger teens for sex. Our teens need to be told that no one has the right to push them into sex. It is their bodies and only they can give permission for someone they can trust to touch them. We have to walk a fine line between caution and making our children overly fearful. We want them to know that sex can be a beautiful experience **with the right**

person. Choosing that right person and that right time is the hard part. We each must take charge of our bodies and our relationships so that no one can persuade us to act in a way harmful to others or ourselves.

As a straightforward, honest parent who is not afraid to talk to your children about anything, you will no doubt be called upon to comment on what you think of masturbation. It is very likely that you will have to bring the subject up. This topic has been, and still is, even more forbidden than sex with a partner. Several years ago, Dr. Jocelyn Elders, then the U.S. Surgeon General, was fired when she expressed her belief that teenagers should be told about using masturbation as a substitute for sex. She believed it was another choice for responsible sex. Teens may talk to each other about masturbation and may want their parents to discuss it with them. Most likely, they have been exploring their body parts since they were small even if you didn't see it happening. When sexual urges happen, they happen, and no amount of wishful thinking will make them disappear. We can be realistic about that and help our children understand that:

1. Sexual urges and bodily changes are normal.
2. Sexual gratification through masturbation is normal, harmless and widely practiced.
3. Masturbation does not cause hand warts, as grandfather's old medical books warned about.

Surveys show that many sexually active teens are using various forms of masturbation to avoid pregnancy and AIDS. Avoidance of sexually transmitted diseases will be discussed in Chapter 7.

As parents, it is our deepest wish to keep our children from all the cruelty and harm we know exists in this big world. Realistically, we also know that our children must, as we did, learn many hard truths on their own. However, we can arm them with every bit of knowledge and love we have to give. "Our children are messengers we send into a future we will never see" (Anonymous). They must discover for themselves how to use our gifts of wisdom and knowledge. We hope they will choose some of our dreams and weave them into their own.

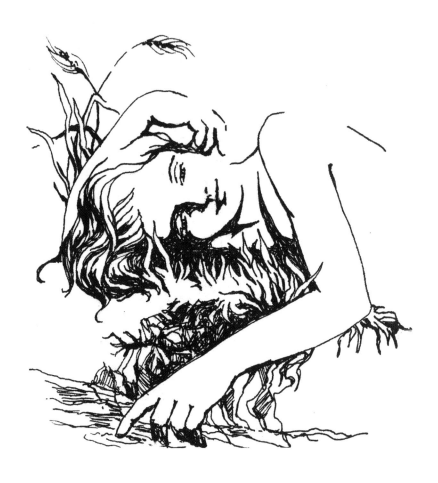

CHAPTER 7

HOW DO WE TALK ABOUT ATTRACTION, AFFECTION, LOVE AND SEX? PARENTS ASK QUESTIONS ABOUT THEIR TEENS' DEVELOPMENT

"By the teenage years, sex education is already too late."
Haim Ginott in **BETWEEN PARENT AND TEENAGER** *(1969)*

INTRODUCTION

As loving parents we want to help our young teens successfully steer through all the stages of growing up, including attraction toward a special person, which may grow into affection and later, into love and possibly a committed relationship. We cannot shield them from all the hurts, temptations and poor choices they are almost sure to encounter, no matter how much we may wish to. Remember when we had these lessons to learn ourselves? We can, however, act as somewhat of an insurance policy for our teens when they encounter hurt or danger. Teens need their parents to be there for them consistently. We can't always be there physically but we **can** let them know that they can rely on us to listen, support them and that we do have their best interest at heart.

Recent surveys show that when we take time to ask teenagers about their opinions, they tell us that they want trusted adults in their lives to help them make important decisions. They may try to look cool and mature outwardly, but inside, this growing up business is very new and scary to them. Our young teenage grandson expressed it well when he stood 6 feet 2 inches tall and told us, "I may look big but I feel tiny on the inside."

Paul Swets, author of *THE ART OF TALKING WITH YOUR TEENAGER* (1995) says, "The way we communicate with our children has an astonishing influence over those children's happiness or ...despair." Research shows an unmistakable link between the breakdown of communication in the home and major social problems such as drug use

55

and drinking, unwanted pregnancies, violent crime and the current increase of suicide among troubled children and adolescents (Berns, 1997).

Whatever mistakes we as parents and caregiving grandparents may have made, we must be doing something right. In a poll done in 1999 for *Time* magazine and TV's Nickelodeon, 1,172 children ages 6 to 14 and 397 parents in 25 cities were interviewed. A strong majority of the children said they felt safe and happy and 79% said they most admired Mom and Dad (Wallis, 1999).

Those admired parents are very likely to have some special parenting qualities that insure that their children feel safe and happy. When they communicate with their teens, it is very likely that they try not to intrude or push their children into "telling them everything." However, they **do** let them know the rules and the consequences. "Be home by 11 o' clock. Call if you have a problem being home on time."

The children of the parents described above have, from the beginning, told their parents where they were going and with whom they were going. These parents know their children's friends because they encourage after-school time at their homes and host parties there. Young friends who visit call these welcoming parents "cool" and even talk to them about problems they can't bring up in their own homes. These parents are not uptight about teenager's first loves or about the sexual urges of their teens. If they followed the child rearing philosophy set forth in the first chapters of this book, these parents most likely feel capable of meeting the new challenges that their dating teens may bring home to them. They have earned the trust and respect of their teens and in return, they can trust that their teens will make wise choices when they are on their own.

The following section consists of questions and answers designed to help parents communicate more successfully with their teenagers. That, as we know, is not an easy task. By the teenage years, values and attitudes toward the world are pretty well set. Often teenagers will experiment and make mistakes, many times without sharing their secrets with us until it becomes obvious to them that they have no way out. We have to trust that our early influence and guidance will stay with them when we are not around. If they have learned love and respect from us they will be more likely to know how to love and respect themselves and others.

QUESTIONS AND ANSWERS

TEENS REACH OUT TO PARENTS AND FRIENDS FOR HELP

Q. I have noticed that our young teen seems to understand more and care more about the family's and his friends' feelings these days. This is a welcome change, but will it last?

A. "Adolescents," according to leading researchers such as L. Steinberg (1993) "make great strides in their development both intellectually and socially in the teen years." They are increasingly able to figure out why people act the way they do as they learn to put themselves in the "shoes" of others, especially friends. They can understand and often want to discuss things like who they are becoming. They are developing more independence and are learning about intimacy and sexuality. They also like to be recognized for their achievements. When you observe a new skill or behavior, let your teen know that you appreciate it. Your encouragement reinforces that desirable behavior which may last for a lifetime.

BEING IGNORED BY A TEEN IS NO FUN

Q. Why does my 14-year old always seems to heading for the door when I try to talk to him. How can we ever have a parent-child talk?

A. Ask yourself, is there real two-way communication going on here? That means an honest exchange of ideas, feelings, and requests between parent and child. If your teen feels that the conversation has tipped over to the parents' side of the argument, ask "Am I steering this in my direction? Am I dominating, being judgmental, negative, or sarcastic?" If so, an apology would be helpful. Otherwise, don't be surprised if your teen heads for the door. Be prepared for reactions from your teen ranging from yelling to sullen, glazed-over eyes, slumped shoulders and few, if any words. If the wall between you seems too hard to break through alone, then you may need to seek out a skilled, qualified counselor to help you and your teen understand one another. (See Appendix C on organizations to help you find a qualified counselor.)

PRIVACY IS A BIG ISSUE WITH TEENS

Q. My young teen used to tell me all about what happened at school, but now I get "Nothing much" as an answer when I ask how the day went. Any suggestions?

A. Privacy becomes very important to young teens and any questions about their experiences may seem like we are prying. Also, sometimes they find it difficult to put their feelings into words, even to themselves. This is especially true during puberty when hormones cause them to be on an emotional roller coaster. If we want our teens to come to us and share what excites them, what scares them, or what makes them laugh or cry, we need to wait patiently until they feel like sharing, not just at our convenience. And sometimes they want us to just let go, without giving the usual advice or unwanted "solutions" we think we owe them as the "wise ones." We can't always fix things but we should always be willing to share and understand. When they are ready to talk to us, it is important to set aside the time even if it means postponing other tasks. Of course, we need to intervene quickly if we feel that our children may be troubled or in danger, even if they do protest that we are ignoring their privacy.

FRIENDS WHO MAY SPELL TROUBLE

Q. How can I be sure my teen's friends are good for him?

A. There is no way to guarantee that our children will pick friends we would choose for them. If we pressure them too much to make "our" choices we may actually drive them further into a harmful relationship. If you've kept communication lines open through your teen's early years and have been a "cool" parent, liked by your child's friends, chances are your child will tend to pick emotionally healthy friends. Sometimes, no matter how cool you've been (meaning children like to come to your house and hang out) your child may still bring a troubled friend to your home. Most likely that friend is being neglected or overly disciplined at home. It is very important that you be cordial and treat that friend with respect. Your teen is watching. Sometimes these friendships break up on their own and sometimes you seem to have "adopted" a child that wants to hang around your house and be part of a friendly family. Even though we can't dictate to our children who will be their friends, we can stick with our parental expectations and rules to help our child and friends stay safe. It does indeed take a village to raise a child.

MY TEEN IS "TOO YOUNG" TO HAVE A GIRLFRIEND/BOYFRIEND

Q. When my young teen says, "I have a girlfriend (or boyfriend) at school," what should I say?

A. Some children around nine or ten or even earlier, like to copy their older role models and say, "She's my girlfriend (or boyfriend) at school." Some parents respond with, "She looks friendly," or "Does she like you?" Parents can think that this is just a cute, early stage of growing up so be careful to avoid laughing or teasing your child or rushing to tell the relatives. It is serious to the child and is a very normal phase of learning about attraction. A child may be attracted to someone of the same sex. Many young adolescents may go through a phase where they feel very close emotionally to a young person of their own sex. This may be a chance for them to "try out" a safe relationship and may last only a short time. Less often, this may be the beginning of a homosexual interest. It can also be a shock to parents to notice what seems like sudden changes in their child whom they still think of as a little kid. Some parents try to postpone the inevitable by ignoring it or forbidding social contacts. That won't work. Teens will always find a way to interact if they want to. They may then hide their relationships and avoid talking about them with you.

When children begin to acknowledge that they have a girl- or boyfriend, they are trying on the idea for size. It's our chance, as parents, to let them know that liking another child in a special way is a normal stage in growing up. Discovering that they can be attracted to someone is very important and the way we react will set up important attitudes, possibly for the teen's lifetime. You might react by saying, "Oh, yes, I know who he is. He has a nice smile," or "Does he like to talk to you?" Later you can suggest, "Maybe he can come over to our house. Would you like to ask him?"

FIRST ATTRACTIONS

Q. My fifteen-year-old boy is definitely attracted to a fifteen-year-old girl in his class. He's mentioned her name, but that's about all I've heard. How can I find out more without being called "nosy"?

A. Your awareness of the importance of your teen's privacy is important. In the situation described, parents are sometimes sorely tempted to launch into "TWENTY QUESTIONS," which often sends teens diving for cover.

59

Do show an interest because you **are** interested and teens really want you to pay attention.

You might say the following, "She sounds interesting. Want to tell me what she's like?" If the answer is "Later," accept that and wait until your teen is ready. Some teens can really get embarrassed if you show too much enthusiasm or interest in their friends, especially in **front** of their friends. A good rule of thumb is to "follow their lead and no pushing from behind." Suggest a fun activity to help you get acquainted. Plan a family picnic or a trip to an amusement park, or allow your teen to plan a party at home, with you in attendance in another room. If you are a "cool" parent, your teen will be happy to introduce you to friends and call on you if the need arises. You may make an occasional appearance to refill the punch bowl. Teens feel safe when they have you nearby. Remember, children sometimes use their parents as an excuse to ask their friends to leave when it was actually your teen who wanted the party to be over.

NO EYE CONTACT

Q. I'm worried. My teenage son is sullen, rarely speaks to us and avoids eye contact when he comes home. What's going on?

A. If your child won't look at you, eyes glazed over and constantly has an expressionless face, take it seriously. This is the behavior of an unhappy teenager. Lighten up on the pressure and seek help from a professional guidance person you trust, one who may have been recommended to you by a reliable source (see Appendix C). Failure to communicate effectively with your teen is a red flag and could signal that a child is in trouble emotionally. When they can't talk to us about their problems and pain, they turn to other, often unhealthy sources. The temptation is to heap more discipline, angry words and restrictions on these often sullen and even disrespectful teens. Sadly, that attitude will only drive them farther away from us.

MIXED MESSAGES BETWEEN TEEN BOYS AND GIRLS

Q. My 16-year old son is confused about how to act toward girls his age. He says that some of his friends think that girls just want to "make out" with guys and don't really want to try and get to know each other as persons. I think these kids are copying what they see on television. On many of the shows they watch, girls and boys act like being sexual is the only important goal. What's going on here?

60

A. You make a good point. Since teens may have only their friends to learn from, the media becomes a powerful outside source, shaping their attitudes and behaviors surrounding sex. Teens may believe what they see on TV and think that the shallow way young people are portrayed in certain comedies is true, that girls are "just out for a good time and that superficial sex is desirable." That, however, is not what we want our children to learn in preparation for adulthood. Furthermore, some notions about the opposite sex which (our) teenagers pick up from their friends, or on the street, turn out to be quite wrong or overly simplified.

Instead, we need to help our children learn that both males and females crave respect, and want to be treated with dignity and compassion at all times. Anything less than that is a way of dehumanizing our relationships and will only bring anger and heartache. No one really wants to be treated like a sex object or play toy, and if we share this with our children early in life, and model it in our homes, they will benefit enormously.

TALKING ABOUT SEX WON'T INCREASE
THE PREGNANCY RATE

Q. I really want to help my young teen learn about responsible sex, but I've heard that giving them all the information is just an open invitation for them to have sex. Is this true?

A. Research in the United States and around the world has shown this **not** to be true. Studies report that when young teens have an understanding about their body and how to protect themselves from pregnancy and sexually transmitted diseases (STDs), they are much less likely to have an unwanted pregnancy or disease (Planned Parenthood, 1998). Girls with high self-esteem who have attended quality childcare classes do better in school and wait an average of two years longer to have a baby. Even for those who have a first baby in their teens, with such classes they usually postpone having a second baby.

Girls often have babies in their teens because they have little hope or many aspirations for other life goals. They need affection, and if they do not get it from a parent or parents, they may seek it from another teenager or an older man who may father their child. The child then becomes the object of their affection. More teens than ever now know how to get birth control devices, yet we have the highest rate of teen pregnancies of any developed country. The teen's feelings about her or himself is the critical factor in whether or not they use birth control or adopt abstinence.

Teenage pregnancy rates are gradually going down in most states. Authorities say that this has to do with not only better information on prevention, but because more parents are talking to their children about the consequences of unwanted pregnancies. More girls are achieving academically and going to college now. Many want to achieve various goals before becoming mothers.

The myth that keeping sex education from teens will reduce unwanted pregnancy is dying out as it should. If you believe that your teen has the right to know about protection from pregnancy and diseases, then go to a good bookstore or library that carries that information. Take your teen to a clinic or a trusted doctor. Planned Parenthood has been advising teens and their parents on these vital subjects for many years and can be trusted to offer the latest information on types of birth control with no pressure. They offer excellent written material and videos that you can preview in their libraries.

THAT TALK WITH TEENS WHO ARE BECOMING SEXUALLY ACTIVE

Q. I'm getting hints that my teen thinks it's time to experiment with sex. Her friends are already. I'm not ready for this! I want to yell "abstinence" but I know the hysterical approach won't work.

A. We are rarely ready for this moment. We discover that the teen's timelines are not ours. You are correct in saying that the hysterical approach won't accomplish your goals, the first of which is persuading your child to listen to you and at least consider your point of view. Hopefully, you've been promoting your viewpoint long before this moment. Whether you believe in abstinence before marriage or want your teen to know all the alternatives, it's indeed very important to let your teen know how you feel. If you have not already discussed it, do it now. Calmly lay out the facts. Avoid tiptoeing around the subjects of abstinence, birth control, unwanted pregnancy and sexually transmitted diseases. Straight talk about serious subjects will earn your teen's respect and always works best even if they clam up and stomp out of the room, which they rarely do at a time like this. They are too interested in what you are about to say. Scare tactics usually backfire. It seems to make the forbidden look more exciting. Also, it tends to make you look like less of an authority since teens have trouble believing that anything will happen to them. Sadly, many teens don't listen until they, or a friend get into difficulty. All you can do is avoid placing blame (that usually shuts doors) and listen to their stories, then offer your own truths and reasons for your beliefs. Give lots of eye contact, keep you voice calm and hope that your child will choose a non-destructive path. Of course, we have to be ready to act in their behalf to keep them out of danger when they lose control. Also, call on school counselors and other advisors who will help if asked.

Keep in mind that we are not their masters, just their guardians and thankfully don't still have the outdated mentality that believed that "children are to be seen and not heard" with punishments such as beatings, being chained and starved if they talked back or disobeyed. It helps to keep in mind that we were once their age. Remember the mistakes we made back then?

If abstinence before marriage is your belief, then say so and suggest that there are ways to be close without actually having intercourse. (See the section on Masturbation, Chapter 5). If they decide against abstinence, and sometimes they won't tell you if you are strongly pro-abstinence, then we hope they can learn where to get help, information and the support they need. It may be hurtful for your teen to choose a different path from yours but the most hurtful part would be if you stopped communicating. If it's too hard to talk about certain areas, see if a close relative or friend can be your stand-in.

A QUESTION ABOUT BIRTH CONTROL

Q. I found birth control pills in my daughter's room while cleaning up. What should I say to her? I was not trying to snoop.

A. Important questions to ask yourself are, "How do I feel about my daughter having sex and what kind of communication have I already established with my daughter?" Lecturing or scolding will not work, no matter how frustrated or shocked you may feel. If communication is good, you can find out what she is doing with the pills. Try not to assume that she is sexually active unless you have already seen signs that this is happening. She may have them for future use. It's important to remember that she is the one in control of her body and ultimately she has to make these very personal decisions. You want her to consider you as her ally and know that you are on her side even if you don't agree with her choices. Parents who come across to teens as the enemy may find that when that very delicate thread of trust and communication is broken, it is difficult if not impossible to mend it. You do want to stress how much you care about her and her health and happiness. Then talk about your deep concern about sexually transmitted diseases which are not prevented by birth control pills. It is very helpful to have good books nearby so that you can share expert information. The book for teenagers, *CHANGING BODIES, CHANGING LIVES* (Bell, 1998) is an excellent choice. Our grandchildren recommend it.

TEENS' PROVOCATIVE QUESTIONS ABOUT SEX

Q. My young teen likes to tease. We've talked about sexuality and never tried to avoid subjects about sex. He asks very personal questions about my sex life. How do I respond?

A. Explain only what feels comfortable for you and give no attention to the teasing, silly behavior. It's your private business, you can explain, just like it will be with your teen when he gets older. Answering serious questions about sex in an honest, general way is helpful but personalized, graphic descriptions are not. You may want to share your experiences growing up as a young teen, describing some funny and embarrassing moments when you felt awkward. Teens really want to hear about their parent's growing up stories. They feel closer to you and also know they are not alone. You know to end the story-telling session when their questions stop and the yawning begins.

PERMISSIVE PARENTS NEED TO SET LIMITS

Q. My teen never wants to tell me where he's going and I worry until he gets home. What should I do?

A. If a parent fails to get regular reports on their young teen's whereabouts, that's being too permissive. Get a full report from them the very first time you let them leave home with a friend or alone. Starting out with safe habits is much easier than trying to impose a limit later on. Be sure you have their destination, a phone number if possible and be clear on the time they will return home. Be prepared to negotiate and stick to your reasonable rules agreed upon by both of you. Most healthy teens will try to talk you out of any rule you make at first. But they're impressed if you are consistent and have logic on your side. If teens know you keep your word, they will test the rules much less. If, however, you waiver and let the rule slide even once, you will have trouble on your hands. It takes twice the effort to establish the rule again and make it stick.

PARENTS DISAPPROVE OF THEIR TEEN'S CHOICE OF BOYFRIENDS

Q. My daughter is attracted to a young man who, I believe, may be harmful for her. She has a mind of her own, and I'm not sure how to protect her.

A. When our children start dating, the biggest protection is the love, caring and good communication we've shown them throughout their young lives. Avoid the tactic, "No, you can't see him anymore," which almost guarantees that she will have to defend him and find a way to see him secretly. Those hidden relationships can be the most harmful.

A better approach is to invite her friend to come home, have dinner, maybe watch TV or play games or anything else that will help your daughter evaluate this special boy. Avoid criticizing him. Chances are that she will see him in a different light as she observes him in various situations. If she doesn't, then at least you will be there for her to confide in and help her learn to make better choices.

A CHILD ASKS, "WHAT IS ORAL SEX?"

Q. I have been waiting to have "the big talk" with my ten-year old. He just asked me, "What is oral sex?" How much should I tell him?

A. Children encounter explicit sexual language on TV, in the movies, in the print media, on the internet and many other places. To them, these are simply interesting words that seem to be very important to adults, so they ask us about them. All questions deserve an honest answer. Try to use correct anatomical terms your child can understand. A good book on physiology or human sexuality can help. Stay calm, avoid lectures or verbal attacks. Each parent has a personal opinion on the moral implications of sex scandals in the media, but too much negative moralizing may cause a child's attention to wander.

WHERE IS MY TEENAGER TONIGHT, REALLY?

Q. I worry when my teenager is out of the house. He tells me where he's going, but I'm afraid he may go elsewhere and get involved in risky behavior with his friends. What can I do?

65

A. We know teenagers can invent all kinds of ways to get where they **really** want to go while telling their parents they are somewhere else. We can't stop all such behavior because we can't follow them around. However, some precautions can be helpful. First, develop honest communication with your child early on, **before** the teenage years. (See Chapter 1 on Communication.) Set up very clear curfew and other safety rules before your child begins to go out with friends. Be sure the penalties for broken rules are understood by your child, and that the penalties are logical and reasonable to fit the offense. For instance, taking away privileges for short periods works well. Be consistent in applying the penalties. Say only what you really will do. Other tips collected from wise parents are:

1. Be sure to get acquainted with the parents of your child's friends. Get their work and home phone numbers.

2. Find out if older siblings or a young adult will be along and decide how responsible you think they are.

3. Know your teen's exact destination and have them call you if they leave for a new destination. If they don't call, call them.

4. Be sure they know the time when they are expected home and if they do come in late, without an emergency related reason, be prepared to take the privileges away that you both agreed on beforehand. Expect this to happen one or two times until your teen believes that you mean what you say.

5. If your teen is caught in a lie, it helps to talk about your sadness that they couldn't trust you enough to tell you the truth. Then decide on a penalty that's logical, e.g., come in earlier next time, no use of the car for a week or whatever works best for your teen. Once the incident is over, refrain from bringing up the subject again. Stay in the here and now.

A parent who is really aware and takes consistent actions concerning their teen's whereabouts will earn the respect of the teen even if there is lots of moaning and complaining.

GRANDPARENTS AS CAREGIVERS

Q. I am a grandparent who has had to take over the parenting role for a young teenage grandchild whose parents will have to be absent for a long time attending a rehabilitation program. I live in a different part of the country and have spent little time

with this child. I worry that I may not be able to be up to supervising my grandchild, and meet the needs of a growing teen. What if she resents me?

A. It can be scary to take on such a big responsibility. You can reach out to many organizations and services which specialize in such work with grandparents who are parenting. You are not alone. According to the Census Bureau, more than one in twenty children are in homes headed by grandparents. Take advantage of the books written on guidance and communication and make use of the suggestions in this book on developing good communication with your grandchild. It is very important to remember to show respect for the child's feelings about his or her parents and refrain from painting a negative picture of them to the child. In most cases, no matter what the parents' problems, the child doesn't need to hear negative opinions from others. If the **child** expresses these, you can be a good and active listener and keep the child's friendship with you intact.

FATHERS NEED TO TALK TO THEIR TEENS ALSO

Q. My divorced husband insists that I be the one to talk to our teenager about everything -- sex, drugs, AIDS, etc. He says it's my job and I can do it better. I believe that he also needs to share in this.

A. You are quite right! A recent report by the National Center on Addiction and Drug Abuse at Columbia University backs you up. As the 1999 study points out, children who have poor relationships with their fathers are 68% more likely to abuse drugs of all kinds than those teens in an average two-parent household. It seems that children have an easier time talking to their mothers, and mothers influence their children's choices three times more than fathers. These findings are not a reason for fathers to get discouraged or give up. Mothers and fathers, divorced or not, have to try extra hard to stay in close touch with their children at all age levels and talk to them many times about the dangers out there. Even if the child seems to ignore you, say it anyway. They hear you when you aren't aware they are listening. Children need both parents to be actively involved in their welfare.

CONSTANT BATTLES WITH MOM
CAN HURT A GIRL AS AN ADULT

Q. Since my 12-year old hit puberty, we have had almost constant battles on almost everything she wants to do -- what she wears, when to go to bed, her choice of friends, on and on. I'm at my wit's end. She was an obedient little child and didn't cause me any problems.

A. As frustrated as you must feel, it is important to step back and look at this problem from your child's perspective as well as your own. Some questions to ask: "Is it important for me to win all the arguments with my child, so she'll know who's in charge?" Does it seem like your daughter is attacking you personally and you have hurt feelings? Do you only show affection when your child does exactly as you say? If so, then you and your child will have a very difficult time ever finding common grounds of agreement. Children, especially teens, have their own preferences and cannot simply adopt yours. They need to practice trying out new ways of dressing, eating, and almost everything else. They need to know you still think that they are acceptable and lovable in your eyes. We get into trouble when we only show affection when our children show us blind obedience (which rarely ever happens anyway). Ask yourself – "Is the behavior I dislike causing my child permanent health or safety problems or violating any laws?" If not, then you may want to watch and wait and be tolerant of behaviors that will probably not last very long anyway. Remember that adolescents are almost compelled to reject some of their parent's values, perhaps only temporarily, to then be able to separate and eventually establish their own values. When we understand this, we can avoid seeing their behavior as lasting forever.

Above all, stay friends while at the same time sticking to your limits for health and safety. Studies show that girls who become alienated from their mothers are more likely to demonstrate delinquent behavior, use drugs and do poorly in school. Girls especially need the nurturing contact of their mothers or another mother figure who never rejects them as a person.

TEEN-AGE GIRLS NEED PARENTS WHO LISTEN

Q. When my young daughter does decide to confide in me, I worry about saying the wrong thing and getting upset at her

opinions. Sometimes I get excited and talk too fast and my teen cuts off the conversations. What should I do if my child says things that shock me yet I still want her to confide in me?

A. Mary Phipher (1994) tells us that "certain kinds of homes help girls hold on to their true lives." Structure and affection are the magic words here. Your daughter needs to feel she can express her feelings and wishes freely, but you also have the right to be honest with her about your feelings. You have a special obligation to share your opinions and beliefs with your child. Because your child knows you love and respect her, she will listen even if it looks to you like her attention has wandered elsewhere. Pipher says, "What holds girls lives in place is love and respect for their parents." If parents disagree with their teen's opinion and believe an idea could be harmful, then that has to be said clearly. A respected parent will be listened to and will be heard.

Perfection is not part of a growing teenager's chief concern. They are into trial and error behavior which, unfortunately involves lots of errors. We adults may not have been given such freedom in the past, so it's difficult to let go with our children. We need to create enough space for them to maneuver as safely as possible and to find their limits. We don't want to encourage disrespect either. If we find that we have been too harsh, or even too permissive, we can offer a friendly apology for past mistakes. Children love to forgive us when we're sincere and then they also learn to apologize to **us** when appropriate.

EARLY AND LATE MATURING ADOLESCENTS

Q. My daughter began puberty early and has a womanly figure at 11 years of age. She has trouble fitting in with her girlfriends who are not so far along: How can I help her feel more comfortable about her maturing body?

A. Early maturing adolescents can have feelings of isolation when they are in a group of friends who are not experiencing bodily changes so quickly. If feelings of low self-esteem develop, your teen may be more likely to get involved with older teens and with deviant activities such as using drugs or becoming sexually active, while developing problems in school. You can help counteract these potential problems by listening attentively and developing good rules and consistent limits. Avoid any hint of teasing, which is humiliating to many young girls. Especially avoid remarking on how "grown-up" he or she looks or pushing adult-looking clothes and makeup on them. Let them make the first move even though you may feel great pride and want to dress them up. Teens are very sensitive to parental pressures. Studies show that the way they see themselves is a critical factor in growing up happily. If parents allow daughters to develop their own comfort level without "pushes" from parents, early maturation may not be as difficult as we anticipate.

TEASING HURTS

Q. My 12-year old daughter is beginning to look physically mature, and boys make loud suggestive remarks, whistle, etc., wherever she goes. She isn't ready to date and is embarrassed by this kind of attention. How can I help her?

A. Pay close attention to her need for protection, expressing your understanding of how uncomfortable it must feel being harassed in this way. Let her know that you will work with her to find a way for her not to be alone if possible in those situations and that she doesn't have to look or speak to anyone harassing her. If it happens at school she can talk immediately to the principal. As she gets older she may feel more able to let the boys know that this kind of attention is unwelcome (Steinberg, 1993).

A BEARD AT TWELVE?

Q. My son is twelve-years old and already has beard growth, voice changes and he looks more like sixteen. He's our oldest and I expect a lot of him even though he still acts like a kid. How much should I expect from him?

A. Early maturing adolescents and their parents often face special problems. We have to walk a fine line because we know young teens want to be treated seriously as they are growing up, yet at the same time they still have children's feelings and behaviors. It can be really confusing. Early maturers have the problem of often being pushed by peers and parents into behaving as if they are older and the teen may try hard to do things they aren't ready for, such as sexual exploration with a peer. This causes frustration and confusion for them and they may act out their feelings in negative ways.

Research shows that some teens later become conformists as adults because they have tried so hard to meet outside expectations, rather than make their own choices. Perhaps the best chance we have as parents to keep communications open with our early maturing child is to be alert to their moods. Avoid making critical or sarcastic remarks about how they frequently change their behavior. Though you can't condone or allow disrespectful or dangerous behavior to continue, you can try to accept where your child is at a given moment and listen to their feelings. If they aren't in a talkative mood you can pick up on their facial expressions and body language and comment, i.e., "I get the feeling you don't want to talk right now" or, "You seem really upset. If you want to talk about it, I'm here to listen." You can talk about a problem of any kind, even if your teen only looks at you. Remember, they are listening even if they don't respond at that moment. You can bring up sensitive subjects if they need to be aired and if you are non-judgmental. Your teen will hear you and probably be glad that you did it. Just don't always expect a response.

If your child looks 16 but is acting like a little kid, let him. Join in and have fun with him. You may find that letting your childlike self out will be a delight for you both.

BODY CHANGES CAN EMBARRASS YOUNG TEENS

Q. My daughter is noticing changes in her body but doesn't talk about her developing breast and pubic hair, though I notice her looking in the mirror. Should I act as if I notice or wait for her to bring it up?

A. Young maturing teens, boys and girls, are often self-conscious about their changing bodies. Hopefully you have talked with her and looked at books, discussing upcoming puberty. If so, it is easy to say, "It looks like your body is growing and changing just as we talked about it." Let her know she is attractive and that every girl goes through these changes. As you bring in books with clear illustrations, it will be easy to assure your teen that nature has a beautiful plan and that all these changes are normal. Boys need to be reassured that their erections, and wet dreams which may come as a surprise, are also quite normal. These changes will be accepted as they get older.

TEENS FEELING PRESSURE TO HAVE SEX

Q. My son is 15 and some of friends are beginning to date, mostly in groups but some are pairing off with girls. He worries about how to ask for a date and what to do if he gets pushed into having sex because his friends are doing it.

A. First of all, you need to assure your son that no one has the right to push sex on him, period. There is no one right age when people first have sexual relations with others. Each person decides this for him or herself. Someone who tries to control a friend like that is not much of a friend. For example, we don't let someone tell us what flavor of ice cream to order or what clothes to wear if we dislike what they suggest. Sex is something like that. Each person's body tells us how it feels, when and where it wants to be touched, what feels good, what's scary or annoying. Parents can help their children to be their own best friend and say "no" strongly when someone is intruding on their space and their bodies.

INEXPERIENCED TEEN IS AFRAID TO DATE

Q. My teen daughter is afraid to date. She has heard too many stories of girls being assaulted by boys on dates. She says she doesn't know what to say to let the boy know that she wants to go slow and not become sexual so quickly or even that she wants to wait until marriage. I want her to have a safe, happy social life. What can I tell her so she can feel more in control of her own body?

A. Growing up today for girls can be confusing and complicated, especially with dating. Girls may feel uncomfortable about how they look or if they will be popular even if they say no to sex. They have heard about date rape and about being "dumped" if they do not have sex. Often, girls don't talk about their feelings for fear of being "uncool" or getting a bad reputation. It is important that your daughter feel that she can talk to you. You can help her feel good about accepting her own comfort level for becoming intimate on a date. Girls often want to discover their sexuality more slowly than boys. They can learn to be in control of their behavior and think ahead before they go on a date. You can encourage your daughter to imagine how she will set the limits she wants her date to observe. If she wants to experience touching but not "go all the way," she can make it clear early in the relationship. If the dating partner doesn't respect her enough to listen, then that date is not the one for her anyway.

VIOLENCE IN TEEN RELATIONSHIPS

Q. My seventeen-year old daughter is dating a boy who shows a lot of jealousy toward her. He doesn't want her to be with any

other friends, or go anywhere without him. I'm worried that he'll cut her off from her family as well. She says she really loves him.

A. The type of jealousy problem you describe is definitely a critical warning sign to heed. It's often a first step to violence later in the relationship. Adolescents are carving out an independent identity. Self esteem is often tied to the success of a relationship with a girlfriend or boyfriend. Your daughter's boyfriend may not be able to share her with anyone else because of a self-esteem problem. This problem could escalate into demeaning language, threats, humiliation, mean-spirited teasing and outright physical violence. If you daughter is feeling low in self esteem, she may not be able to leave this relationship, or she may feel afraid of retaliation. She may need your help to reject this kind of treatment and to report it to the police if necessary. It is vitally important to talk to teens about this **before** the problem actually occurs.

If her boyfriend feels uncertain about himself and inadequate about his ability to have a successful relationship, he may believe that having a partner who is obedient and submissive to his abuse will help him feel more adequate. If your daughter refuses to go along with this kind of treatment, her boyfriend may feel threatened and betrayed as if the one he cares about is withdrawing her support. An abusive partner may try to force compliance in any way possible, not realizing that love and loyalty cannot be commanded; nor will it grow when a partner is degraded. It is important to caution your daughter that abusive people can become dangerous if they feel threatened. Seek counseling and legal help if necessary. There are excellent and experienced resources available. (See Appendix A). If attention is not given to stopping abuse in the teen years, violence is likely to occur again with others in later years. Abusive relationships in teen years along with feelings of powerlessness and denial can carry over into adulthood. Victims in these relationships usually suffer from low self-esteem (Hildebrand, 2000). There are agencies and professionals ready to help (see Appendix C).

Often a teen in this kind of trouble will distance him or herself even more from parents and friends. Be alert to the signs and talk with your teen often. It is wise to seek out counseling as soon as possible. There is much professional help available in this area. We do not have to face these problems alone. Each city has a form of Domestic Violence Hotline and often they are printed in the first page of local telephone books. It's wise to keep that number close at hand.

WILL TEENS BECOME PROMISCUOUS?

Q. I worry that today's teenagers are out of control and that my adolescent will be overly influenced by peers to act the same way and become promiscuous.

A. It's easy to become frightened when we listen to the news. The media tends to report all the bad news and to exaggerate. The good news is that for several years, surveys on teenage attitudes tell us that the majority of today's teens say that fidelity and honesty are very important in relationships with sexual partners (Conger, 1977). They also say they dislike promiscuous sex or when anyone is pressured or threatened to have sex. They believe that young people should understand about their responsibilities to each other before deciding to have sex. They would also like to have long term emotional, affectionate relationships and commitments. Of course, all teens are not this responsible, so talking with your child is very important.

A DAUGHTER'S FIRST SEXUAL RELATIONSHIP

Q. My teenage daughter has confided in me that she had sex with her new boyfriend. She is quite upset, afraid of what I would say. She seems to care a lot about him but doesn't want her friends to know. How can I help her?

A. It is important that she felt trusting enough to reveal her secret to you. Your daughter's fear of the disapproval of her peers is not unusual for girls today. Boys are given much more acceptance for engaging in sex. Studies report that girls feel "afraid, worried, embarrassed and guilty" after first intercourse. Generally, girls are much more emotionally tied to their sexual experiences than boys are (Sorenson, 1973). Let your daughter know that you understand how she feels and that her feelings are very important. She needs to ask herself if she feels comfortable or does she want to wait until she is older to continue to have sex. Can she discuss it with the boy? Does she know about having responsible sex and do they protect themselves every time? Does she know if they are both free of sexually transmitted diseases through testing?

You do not have to encourage sexual activity but you can let your daughter know she can talk to you and that you will support her as she works out her answers. If you as a parent are not there at these critical

74

times, or are judgmental, your teen will never come to you with sensitive subjects again. This means their decisions will be much harder to make and sometimes, disastrous. Being willing to hear about a teen's real situation, as unpleasant as that may be, is much preferred over silence between you.

TEEN BOYS AND GIRLS VIEW SEXUALITY DIFFERENTLY

Q. I've noticed that my two teenagers, a girl and a boy, are having very different experiences in being introduced to their sexuality.

A. You have observed a very important point about your teens. We may tend to think that girls and boys think alike, but researchers have noted not only hormonal differences, but also social expectations that play a big role as well. Boys are very likely to become sexual through masturbation and often discuss it with their friends early on. They understand what orgasms are before they find a partner. Their early partners are likely to be short term, and "scoring" is very important at this stage (Carns,1973). On the other hand, girls attach a great deal of emotion and intimacy to their first sexual experience which is usually with a partner they would like to stay with. Since pregnancy is a big concern for girls, being more cautious and wanting to remain with the first sexual partner is much more important for girls. Girls who have not had a strong, healthy relationship with a father often look for older young men who will love and take care of them.

IS MY BOY A HOMOSEXUAL?

Q. I am the father of a twelve-year old son. I recently accidentally saw my son being sexual with his male peer. Is this a sign that he is homosexual?

A. Not necessarily. Most adolescents engage in some sexual activity with their adolescent peers. Perhaps as much as one-third of boys experience an orgasm through sexual activity with another male (Kinsey, Pomeroy, and Martin, 1948). In certain middle eastern countries, homosexual behavior between males is accepted before these males are able to marry and then have heterosexual activity. Boys, like girls, like to explore at times but over 90% eventually develop heterosexual relationships exclusively. About 3% become exclusively homosexual (Michael *et al*, 1994). Stay calm and respectful of your teenager's choices. You will not be able to change their preferences for the same or opposite sex (Kinsey, 1948). In some cases these preferences include both the same and opposite sexes.

Research is pointing to biological as well as environmental causes for one's sexual preferences. Since we do not choose our preferences, we want our children to know we support and love them as human beings no matter what their sexual orientation.

CAN HOMOSEXUAL TEENS CHANGE THEIR SEXUAL ORIENTATION?

Q. Why won't counseling and education change my son's mind about being a homosexual?

A. This question has been asked many times by parents. Researchers are just now beginning to get some idea of what factors are involved in sexual orientation. The evidence is pointing to both biological and environmental reasons (Green, 1980; 1987). Medical and psychiatric practitioners have stopped looking at homosexuality as a disease. It's not a condition that a person decides to adopt upon awakening one morning. Nature creates variety in all things and humans are no exception. It is now thought that homosexual preferences may start even prenatally when the fetus is exposed to certain hormones at various times as the brain develops (Savin-Williams, 1988). It is also possible that the tendency to be a homosexual or heterosexual may be inherited. It's important to remember that causes for human behavior are many and complex. It will always be difficult to attach a formula to the causes of homosexual behavior. But it is important to remember that education, counseling, or harassment is not going to change a person's sexual orientation. Even if some individuals conform outwardly to social expectations, their true sexual orientation is not likely to change.

WHY HAVE SEX EDUCATION IN SCHOOLS?

Q. Does sex education in schools help kids? My teenager complains that the teacher doesn't know very much.

A. As the years go by we are gathering more information on what kind of sex education in schools is most useful. Asking students is one very good way to plan helpful courses. First of all, it seems that just talking about sex, or about differences in males and females and the dangers of having sex does not deter teens from trying sex. Why? Teens will discover their sexuality, no matter who tries to discourage them so why not be helpful rather than be a hindrance to them in their search for their own realities and feelings.

The use of the following principles concerning sex education are seen as lowering rates of teenage pregnancies:

1. It is important for young adolescents to learn early about sex, birth control and pregnancy as well as the emotional side of sex. Teenagers need to learn about making choices, being assertive about their feelings (when to say no), and learning about self-responsibility and resisting peer pressure.

2. Having contraceptive and pregnancy prevention information readily available where teens can get them easily is very important. This can be done in combination with school and community-based clinics. This helps to ease the embarrassment teens feel when they can't talk to parents. Teens need a reliable source of information they can go to.

There has been public resistance to school-based clinics, but research shows that clinics and school counselors drastically cut teen pregnancy. Parenting Education classes in schools are also of great benefit to teens and pre-teens. Domestic violence and teenage pregnancy rates go down when teens take such classes (Peraino, 1998; Tyree et al., 1991). The rates of teen pregnancies are much lower in other industrialized countries which have mandatory parenting and sexuality classes compared to the high rate of teen pregnancies in the U.S. (Jones, et al., 1987; Westoff, 1988). It is clear why there is such a difference between the U.S. and other countries. We have much less sex education in our schools and it is not a required subject. We send mixed messages on abstinence to our youth while the media and advertisers promote sexual titillation for profit. We withhold birth control protection and information. While some parents can't or won't be honest with their children about sexual issues, those parents who are, find that there is also resistance by some citizens and politicians to giving our young people the facts they need to know. There is resistance to allowing the schools and clinics to educate teens. We know how to lower teenage pregnancy rates and sexually transmitted diseases. Our teens know that there are answers. It is our responsibility to see that they get them.

CHAPTER 8

NO EASY ANSWERS:
MORE QUESTIONS AND ANSWERS

We dream of moments when our teenagers stop and listen to our words of wisdom or when they bring their friends home to meet us and we like them! After all, aren't we the ones with life experience who could so easily steer them around the dangerous pitfalls if they would but listen? And what about those nightmare times when they stay out too late? They may tell us our ideas about sex are old-fashioned or announce that they are pregnant long before they are ready for such awesome responsibility.

It's so easy to love and enjoy our teens when they are behaving their angelic best. However, they need our love and understanding far more when they are at their most unlovable. Our first instinct may be to sit them down and "talk some sense into them" or let them know that they can come back home when they are willing to follow the house rules! That happens far too often. As a result, many of those children are wandering the streets as prostitutes. Others are on drugs or are selling them and will soon be on their way to jail. Most teens try to be independent even though, most of the time, they haven't had the experience or maturity to figure out what that means. They might never admit it but they need our love and support the most when we might feel like giving it the least. If you want your teen to respect you, stay cool headed with a calm and steady attitude, free of blame, judgment or ridicule. Remember the good communication rules you read in Chapter One. Also remember that **you** are the parent and have control over what goes on in your house as well as the legal and moral responsibility for your teen, no matter how they behave. Someone has to stay cool and you need to be the one. Your teen will feel safer that way even if they do complain loudly or look disgusted. Not giving up on our children is the greatest gift we can give them during these times. These may be the hardest moments you will have as a parent but you are capable and can meet the challenge. Your child is watching you.

The following questions may be new to you. Chances are, many of us would never have thought of asking our parents these questions when we were teens. Today's teens do not hesitate to ask their friends frank, straight forward questions about any subject. They would prefer to ask trusted adults if the adult is comfortable with it. That means you as a parent may have to start a conversation about subjects dealing with sexual behavior, birth control and pregnancy to break the ice. We have been given some positive news about recent studies according to the Center for Disease Control (CDC) (*Newsweek*, 2000.). The number of teens who have had intercourse is at 48%, down from 54% in 1991. Fifty-one percent of teens in a large research sample from "Project Reality" in Illinois said that it is possible to control sexual urges as opposed to 3.5 percent who answered "never possible" (*Newsweek*, *ibid.*). The use of condoms and the pill seem to be more acceptable than ever before, with 57% of sexually active teens reporting that they use condoms. Teenage girls report that 44% prefer the pill and 38%, condoms (CDC, 1991). However, we still have a long way to go. More than half of the 905,000 teen pregnancies in 1996 resulted in births. Three million teens (1 in 4) who are sexually active get a sexually transmitted disease every year. The Guttmacher Institute reports that an increasing number of teens seem to believe that "oral sex" is not real sex, although we know that some STDs are transmitted that way, too.

The National Center for Health Statistics (2000) has noted that teen pregnancies are going down. Not dramatically, but the trend is in the right direction and researchers say it's partly because parents and educators are taking an active role in talking to children about their sexuality and the responsibilities that go with it. As our children grow we tend to talk less with them about these crucial areas. As they begin to look like adults, they need our guidance even more. Continue to observe closely, ask clarifying questions and listen when they need us. That's what our grandchildren tell us to do for them. It is hoped that when children need our help, nothing they say or do is too shocking for us to help them deal with it.

MORE QUESTIONS AND ANSWERS

BORED OR LONELY TEENAGERS CAN TURN TO SEX

Q. My thirteen-year old daughter is beginning to look at boys. I work full time. As a single mom, I haven't had as much time to

be with her as we used to have. How can I help her avoid a sexual relationship too early and perhaps an unwanted pregnancy?

A. Although 85% of pregnant teenagers have unwanted pregnancies, some girls intentionally plan to have their babies, even though they may not admit it even to themselves. Young teens we have interviewed over the years and others quoted in studies said that they wanted a baby to love and to take care of, someone who would think that their Mom was special and needed by the baby. What can be done under such circumstances?

Take time to have fun with your daughter. Get her involved in sports, a hobby, or clubs, or any wholesome community activity that appeals to her. Go with her if she chooses to help her get started. Let her know that you really want to be with her, even if the time available is limited. Girls who are given loving attention, and who spend time with their families in positive ways, develop a high sense of self worth and self esteem. Studies show that girls that get along well with their mothers get into less trouble as they grow into teens (Papp, 1999). These girls usually want to stay in school and prepare for a career that fits their interests and talents. Having a baby is seen by them as something to think about in the future when life is stable and, hopefully, when they have a reliable partner and can provide for their child economically. Babies grow up better that way as the research continues to tell us (Wolf, 1996). Do explain to your budding adolescent that bringing a baby into the world is a serious responsibility. Also, young girls' bodies are not mature yet (neither are their brains, we're learning now), and the chances of the teen mother and baby having early health problems is much greater. Teen parents who cannot finish their education are likely to stay at the poverty level. Talk about and actually work out a budget for a family of two or three so your teen will know that her allowance isn't going to make it. Let her know you cannot be regarded as an unlimited donor.

If your teen, boy or girl, knows another teen who has gone through pregnancy, that's a good opportunity for your teen to observe the problems that come up after their baby is born. If you see a similar story on TV or at the movies, discuss it together. Remind your teen that the demands of the baby are always there. Some school parenting classes have an assignment requiring teens to bring a doll home with them called, "Baby Think It Over" (1999) that requires 24-hour care for a weekend. A computer in the baby records how it has been treated and the students' grades depend on their good parenting behavior. This doll has persuaded many a teen out of early parenthood. It takes a mature adult to handle parenthood well and even then, as we know, it's tough.

We know a family whose 13-year old daughter was sure she wanted a baby. The parents' protests fell flat, but when she watched a real home birth and babysat for a baby and toddler overnight (down the street) she was very clear that she didn't want to have a baby until much later. Chalk up another one for "Experience is the best teacher."

CAN GUILT HELP KEEP TEENS OUT OF TROUBLE?

Q. Does good old fashioned guilt help teens avoid pregnancy? My mother thinks it does.

A. It is tempting to wish we could go back in time when teens were frightened by adults about trying any sexual behaviors (especially girls) for fear of their getting pregnant and being seen as social outcasts or being labeled as "morally loose." The world has changed and our new understanding of how shame and guilt works shows us why the old approaches aren't working as well as some had hoped. When we say "Don't do that" it tends to spotlight that behavior as "forbidden fruit" and makes it more exciting for kids to try it. It gives attention to the very behavior we are trying to discourage. Remember when trying to shame your preschoolers into responsible behavior didn't work, but praising them and building their self esteem with positive attention did? The same principle applies when they are teens exploring the more adult world of sexuality. Research done in the nineteen eighties (Gerrard, 1987) on the subject of guilt and sex shows that those who feel especially guilty about having sex will most likely have less sex, but when they do have it, they often don't use birth control. Why? Because they don't want their partner to see them as prepared and to think they are morally loose. If teens stayed within a peer group who believed in abstinence, they would be more likely to say "no" to sex. However, if they lose the protection of such a group and have sex, they are less likely to use contraceptives. They trust in luck to protect them, but that rarely works.

IT'S NOT EASY BEING A MALE AT ANY AGE

Q. What can I tell my son about the responsibilities surrounding sex and possible fatherhood?

A. Boys have been getting confusing messages for a long time since women began questioning old roles. On one hand, boys get the message

81

from traditional society that they have to be strong, the Rock of Gibraltar, the "take action man," the main breadwinner, and oh, yes, hold in their feelings and take care of things. They are told that if you work hard you can have it all. On the other hand, they hear the new message from women that says, "Show your soft side. Talk about feelings, and it's O.K. to cry." They are being asked to share the housekeeping and childcare chores equally and get used to the idea that women also bring home a paycheck. The old ways of taking charge are now being labeled as "being dominant." Flirting can now be labeled as sexual harassment and if a girl friend gets pregnant, an absent father can be found and legally required to pay his share of child support. These are all topics that today's boys should be aware of and understand.

Young men need to know that women appreciate it when they show and talk about feelings, when they help with family chores, when they baby-sit and play with young children and especially when they think carefully about taking responsibility for their behavior, including sexual behavior. Boys have all kinds of questions to ask about their strong sexual and loving feelings toward another and how to handle them. In today's world, your boy will already have lots of questions. Your job is to create an atmosphere where he will feel comfortable and ask **you** his questions. When that happens, it is one of the greatest compliments he can give you. Sharing innermost questions openly, whether it's "How do I know when to let someone I like know it?" or "Why do I have wet dreams?" you will be challenged to come up with answers you might not have thought about for a long time. At least your teen knows you are paying attention. It's also O.K. to say, "You know, son, that's one I don't know the answer to. Let's see if we can find that one in a book or ask an expert who does know." Honest answers are very comforting to children and they usually know when we try to fool them.

It's a good idea to collect some books and pamphlets about matters that concern teens about sex and do some homework if you are a little rusty on all of this. The latest information on birth control, sexually transmitted disease prevention and much more is available in libraries, clinics, and bookstores.

As parents we have been in training all these years, partly for this very crucial time to help launch our child into adulthood. Your chance might only come once. Be prepared. Know where the agencies are in your community (See Appendix C: Advocacy Information for Families and their Children) and which ones specialize in family planning and health. Then

82

see that your teen gets there after the two of you have decided the course of action you both think is best.

One health service agency, Circulo de Hombres, in San Diego, California, actively helps young teen boys get their priorities straight. They have four goals for the young men who belong.

Young men of honor:

1. Keep their word.
2. Hurt no one.
3. Take responsibility for their actions.
4. Are a positive example for others.

Jerry Tello says of this organization's goals, "Men must be waiting on both sides of the bridge to show the young men the true way of respect, responsibility and dignity. We must first be responsible for our actions before we can expect responsibility from them." We as parents, pass the torch from one generation to the next and it is an awesome but wonderful responsibility.

SPECIAL WAYS TO GET THROUGH TO TEENS --
BREAKING DOWN WALLS.

Q. Try as I will, I can't seem to master the art of having a calm conversation with my teen children. We usually end up in a shouting match with slammed doors and no resolution to the argument at hand. Are there any formulas that work?

A. Teenagers are often quite talented at pushing our buttons. That's one way they can feel they've "won" and perhaps convince themselves that it soon will be time to leave the nest. What we are looking for is a win-win situation where you **both** walk away with your sense of self-respect intact.

A great deal of the success comes in how we present our side of it. Pete Desisto, Director of the Cooperative Learning Institute (1996) suggests some useful techniques. He says, "Give them voice and choice." The following are his suggestions paraphrased:

1. Use a calm voice whenever possible. No shouting or bossy tones.
2. Make good use of humor (not laughing at your teen, but with them) so that they know you are not so emotionally tied to your point of view that you can't see both sides.

3. Rephrase the main points they make in the discussion to be sure your are hearing your children correctly and that they are hearing you.
4. Show a "how can I help" attitude rather than jumping to a conclusion and blaming them. Listen to all sides before drawing conclusions.
5. Pay attention without allowing your mind to wander to the TV (which should be shut off) or the newspaper lying nearby.
6. Move the discussion along and get to the important points. Irrelevant talks tend to frustrate, confuse and doom a helpful solution from being born.
7. Give gentle eye contact. No glaring please.
8. Avoid invading your teen's physical space. Knock on the door and ask permission to come in as you would like done for you.

As loving, responsible parents we never give up trying to communicate and help our children succeed as human beings, from before birth until we die. Let's always keep in mind that we are **all** trying to do our best at any given moment, even if later we wish we'd chosen another course of action. And remember, it's never too late to say, "I'm sorry. Let's try again to solve this one." Then trade hugs and plan a way to have some fun! You've earned it.

AM I REALLY IN LOVE, MOM?

Q. My daughter thinks she's in love with her boyfriend and asks me, "Is this real love?" What do I tell her?

A. This is a tough one to answer. It helps a lot if your teen has observed you and your mate in a successful relationship. We now know it is possible to love someone in many ways. Teens, in the midst of infatuation and sexual attraction may call that "in love" without an awareness that this feeling may well be temporary and not the foundation on which to base a long term relationship. In addition to being in love, successful marriages are based on compatibility and other factors. We give our college students a long questionnaire to fill out at home which includes almost all the areas of marital and partner relationships one can think of. Many young people believe that all things will work out magically if two people just love each other enough. Let's be sure to help them know that there is much more involved when two people merge their lives. The following list may help (not necessarily in order of importance):

84

1. Does your partner want as many good things for you as for him/herself? Does he/she behave as if they really believe that?

2. Can you tell each other anything you feel is important without feeling scared or embarrassed and can you do so while respecting each other's feelings?

3. Can you trust your partner to do what he/she says they'll do, in a timely manner or explain why they can't if something gets in the way?

4. Do you enjoy being with this person with a group of friends or relatives? Are you proud to introduce your partner? Does your partner seem to genuinely like people? Does your partner also like to spend time on his/her own occasionally?

5. Do you feel safe and secure with this person?

6. Is the person able to make plans and carry them out to support him or herself financially? It helps if they have shown they can do this already.

7. Is this person a good listener who respects your opinions but isn't too timid to express his/hers as well and to work out compromises when needed?

8. Can your partner say "I'm sorry" or "I made a mistake" and mean it?

9. Can you both listen to the other when you discuss your sexual preferences and be respectful of each other whatever they may say they want or don't want when being intimate? Do both of you want to use birth control? Will you both be checked out for sexually transmitted diseases?

10. Consider the relationship that each partner has with his/her parents. How does the boy treat his mother and the girl treat her father? And how do these parents treat their children? This can often give us a good idea of how the young couple will treat each other over time.

11. If there is a problem which calls for the help of a professional, how does your partner feel about seeing someone who could help, like a counselor?

12. Do you both feel the same way about moral and religious issues, drugs of all kinds, legal and illegal and about having babies?

13. Do you share most values on politics, sex, religion, and money?

These are all critical areas that too often get lost in the romantic moment when partners first fall in love, yet they need to be discussed and dealt with early in a relationship. We know that people have a hard time changing their basic values and behaviors and it's better to look for the qualities you want in a partner early on, and talk about your concerns together, hoping then that there will be less heartache later.

TEEN PARTNERS WHO DISAGREE
ABOUT THE USE OF BIRTH CONTROL

Q. My older teenage daughter has let me know that her new boyfriend doesn't like to use condoms and often "forgets." He says it's too much trouble and feels weird. They've both been tested for sexually transmitted diseases, but I worry that she will get pregnant. Why is it so difficult to get this across to him?

A. That's an age old question that causes parents and partners a lot of stress. We know that younger teens especially seem to avoid use of contraceptives even if they have no moral objections to them. Center for Disease Control studies show that if a teenager does not use birth control, she will most likely be pregnant within a year (*Newsweek*, 2001). There are probably as many reasons for this attitude as there are couples. Some of the major ones have to do with inconvenience. Suddenly, it's time to have sex and neither partner is prepared. If drugs or alcohol are involved, the rational part of the brain is not functioning well either. Some young men don't think it's "macho" and complain that it takes away sensitivity. Some girls don't want to look "loose" by carrying a condom and appearing to have planned it all ahead of time. A girl is less likely to assert herself and insist that a condom be used for fear of angering her boyfriend and risk losing him.

These are reactions we can predict for many teens. How can parents best head off these attitudes for their children? As with all the subjects you discuss with them as they are growing up, from being careful in crossing the street to saying "no" to drugs, preparation for safe sex is another subject that can't be ignored. We must be able to teach our children the important facts that will protect them when they are older and when they decide to have sex. If we withhold knowledge, we have cheated them out of essential information for successful living. Your parental influence will help them anticipate the problems ahead. They need to learn to envision problem situations and think about how to stay safe **before** they find themselves in a dangerous or awkward moment. At that moment they may not have time to think about what's best for them. It's hard for teens to say "no" to sexual feelings when they are new at it and impulse controls are not well developed. They need to practice what to say. Some teens will even role play with you if you suggest that you play the part of their date. For instance, you might say, "What if your boyfriend said, 'You'd better have sex with me or I'll know you don't really like me.'" Your teen might then say, "I like you, but I'm not ready to have sex now. I need to feel really comfortable with it first and I'm not sure when that will be," or "I'm saving it for marriage."

An important step for your daughter is to be sure that the young man has all the necessary information such as pamphlets, videos and talk with professional healthcare workers. She can be encouraged to let him know that her parents are really concerned also.

If the boy insists, she needs to know it's O.K. to say she wants to go home or calls you at home to pick her up, whatever the circumstances. She should have money for cab fare as well. She can make it clear also that if sex is planned it will be with the use of birth control! If the boyfriend is still unwilling to have safe sex, you can ask your daughter just how important her health is to her partner? Is he willing to put them both at risk? Is this the kind of partner she wants to be with? If he respects her and treasurers her, he'll use a condom. She needs to take charge of her body. Be specific when you talk to your teen. They understand clear messages and are then much better prepared to anticipate and discover ways that they can stay in charge of themselves and their feelings.

WHAT'S THE BEST BIRTH CONTROL?

Q. How do I help my teen learn best about the safest birth control methods?

A. Many parents believe that it is better to give their teen truthful information about safe sex. Parents need to discuss with their young teens how they feel about teen sexual activity and why. Honest discussions are what's important here. Even though you may have talked about birth control or your teen may have read and talked with his/her friends about this, it is very important to discuss it thoroughly. Consult your own physician, or qualified staff in a public or private health clinic who can give your teen expert advise on the best birth control methods and the correct way to use them. County health departments are a good place to start if you are just beginning to look. The following is a general summary of some of the most commonly used methods. A 1997 report of the Alan

Guttmacher Institute states that 54% of the women who began having sex in the 1990's had partners who used condoms, a big increase from previous years.

For teen girls who want more control there are birth control pills, the most popular method, and female condoms. Female condoms have been improved. They also cover the outer genital area and help protect against sexually transmitted diseases.

Other methods such as the IUD, diaphragm, with or without spermicidal jellies are used less frequently by teens, especially younger ones. Injections or Norplant have become increasingly popular (Wingert, 1998). For complete information, consult a clinic, physician and/or Planned Parenthood.

The rhythm method, where intercourse is avoided during the fertile time of the month, is very unreliable and overly complex for teens to try to use successfully.

It can't be stressed enough how important it is for parents to listen to their young teens when you both feel ready to discuss birth control methods if that is your belief. You are building the sense of trust and safety they need for this unfamiliar part of their lives. Teens can obtain birth control information without your knowledge or permission and most will find a way, unless you are there to help them sort it all out and decide when and if they are ready. Your support and attention at this time will help to ensure that they will come to you with problems they don't have to hide. As stated above, current statistics show that the rate of teenage pregnancies has been on the decline since the mid-nineties (*Newsweek*, 2000). Many experts believe this is due to the fact that parents and educators are doing more to help their teens understand all the alternatives available to them.

WOMEN CAN BE IN CHARGE OF THEIR BODIES AND OF BIRTH CONTROL

Q. How can I help my daughter understand that females can be in control of birth control use? What can I say that will help her feel at ease since we haven't talked much about the alternatives?

A. You are certainly wise to let your daughter know that she can be in charge of her own body. If the young man respects her and also wants to have a successful relationship, he will cooperate. If not, she must decide if she is dating an irresponsible male who doesn't have her welfare at heart. Too often, men in their 20's and older impregnate teen girls and leave them to be single moms. Explain to your daughter that there are very definite steps she can take to be in charge and to keep herself safe:

1. She can insist that they both be tested for HIV/AIDS and use a condom and other barriers for oral sex specified in the literature about sexually transmitted diseases. Then go back for tests again in six months, in case the virus might have gone undetected the first time around. Public health clinics or private health care will do these tests and the results are confidential.

2. Your daughter can have condoms available at all times. Some girls and women don't like to seem prepared for fear it will make them look overly eager or "loose." But getting a life-threatening sexually transmitted disease or becoming pregnant are much greater threats.

3. She can buy female condoms which are carried by most pharmacies. They are slightly more expensive. If used correctly, they are quite reliable, but not quite as reliable as male condoms. Usually that is because the woman doesn't use them as directed. Used correctly, female condoms allow the woman to stay in control. They also cover the outer areas of the vagina which offers better protection against some sexually transmitted diseases or parasites.

ABSTINENCE

Q. How can I talk about abstinence so that my young teen will listen and understand the risks of early sex?

A. Abstinence has gotten a bad reputation among many teens. Perhaps it's because parents, teachers, or others may have presented the idea in a stern lecture and so teens tuned them out automatically. Even so, more teens consider abstinence to be a good choice and plan to save sex for marriage and/or that one person they want for their life partner. It certainly simplifies their lives in some ways and gives them the chance to carefully consider who they want as an intimate partner before committing to a serious emotional relationship.

Presenting the idea of abstinence to your teen can be done in a relaxed way, which makes it more likely that they will seriously consider it in a more favorable light. Remember that the "don't" word is like dangling the temptation to try sex in front of a teen. Let your teen know that national statistics show that the majority of teens are not choosing to have sex. If they do however, they need to be very aware of the consequences of an unwanted pregnancy and of bringing another human being into the world. If the choice is to keep the baby, there are questions about the parents staying together, perhaps interrupting their education, having no way to support the child and a whole host of considerations which young teens will not think of on their own.

A number of physicians and other healthcare professionals suggest that teens be advised of the following when considering abstinence or other alternatives (Hatcher, 1996):

1. Decide what you **both** feel about sex, when you are in a good mood, clear-headed and sober. (Maybe as you take a walk.)
2. Decide what sexual activities are O.K. with you and discuss these with your partner.
3. Let your partner know, **in advance**, what you will **not** do.

If your lines of communication have been kept open through the years, you can provide your teen with good information that will give them a head start on making wise choices.

CHAPTER 9

THE CHILDREN ARE WATCHING

From the moment babies are able to focus, they fix their gaze on the closest person meeting their immediate needs of food and closeness. We wait for that moment when we smile at them and they smile back. Mother Nature makes sure that babies pay attention to the cues they need to find the caregiver with the food. Whether we are aware of it or not, that watching never stops. Children, for survival, have to learn how to become mature human beings. To do that their gaze is forever fixed on us, their parents.

It might be argued that the adolescent stage is an exception and the last thing most teenagers want is to be caught watching a parent. Yet they do watch us with great interest. They may try hard to conceal it, because they are trying so hard to break away and become independent. We may not get invited into their world or even thanked for our efforts until later in their young adulthood when they do feel separate and competent out on their own. A few lucky parents are allowed to be included in their children's inner-sanctum world throughout their growing years but it seems to be uncommon. Growing up, separating from parents and gaining independence from parents is a normal process. We know it is another of those phases we've lived through successfully and as adults, we can step back and wait for our children to also become adults. Our patience is usually rewarded if we can keep the lines of communication open.

A child's ability to grow up successfully depends so much on what they learn from us as they watch what we do more than what we say. Parents have the awesome responsibility of being the most helpful models they can be. It is well known that teens create their own world by internalizing the examples parents, friends, teachers and others set for them daily. Teens are, in many ways, in charge of who they are becoming. They choose what they give their attention to. Many parents, the authors included, assumed that we as parents were simply competing with the other influences in our teen's life, and that our teens were just as likely to tune us out.

91

Not so, says reliable research coming out in recent years. In 1996, a Roper Starch Survey reported that 50% of the survey's sample of teenagers who are sexually active say they would have liked to have a talk first with their parents about sex. Those who do, tend to delay first intercourse longer.

In *THE POWER OF ABSTINENCE* (1990), Kristine Napier points out that parents have much more power than they realize. Teenagers are likely to postpone intercourse until later in life if:

1. "Parents stay involved with their children's lives and help them dream for the future; and
2. Lines of communication are kept open; and
3. There are clear guidelines on reasonable and consistent limits, enforced fairly."

Using the above guidelines sends a signal to teens that their parents are taking their own power seriously but not abusing it.

The Henry J. Kaiser Foundation (1966) sponsored a survey which included 1,510 teens, ages 12-18. Approximately half or more of the teens wanted more information on birth control and sex earlier in their lives. They especially wanted more accurate information from their parents. Three-fourths of the teenagers reported that their parents had talked to them about sex but left out information on birth control and sexually transmitted diseases. Teens are very much aware that the information is out there and if their parents don't help them find it, they'll ask someone else who may be less qualified. Sean Daniels, producer-director, who has influenced some wildly popular teenage films said, in a TV interview, that whether we like it or not, "The reality of teenage life is R-rated."

The message is clear. Children want our approval and our wisdom. If we ignore their calls for help, we have lost golden opportunities to be there for them when they need us. Parents too often fail to recognize what is **real** in their children's lives. We continue to hold on to our fantasies for them. Once again, surveys report that teens have different priorities than their parents think they do. A recent survey done by Students Against Drunk Driving and Liberty Mutual Insurance Company found teenagers to be more concerned with drinking and driving and teen suicide, while their parents worried more about car accidents and casual sex. Fifty percent of parents thought their child would not drink and drive, but 21% of the teens said they had done so.

It is disturbing to see such large reality gaps between teens and their parents. Listening skills and involvement by parents are the essential ingredients. Teen marketing expert Irma Zandle, who tracks "under 30 trends", tells us that young people say, that today more than ever, parents are their role models. Listen closely, parents. **Children want the truth and they want to hear it from you.**

The good news is – parents are beginning to "get it"! **It is O.K. to talk about sex with our children.** Full-page ads in newspapers and magazines now boldly tell us to "Talk to Your Kids About Sex." In our youth the word "sex" only appeared in professional publications. The ads

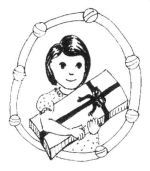

are a good start, but we need more than slogans to get us through. The "Just Say No" campaign failed to slow down drug use in teens. More than any slogan, more than any advice from an organization, more than any sex manual, your child needs **you**. They need your undivided attention. (The television and other distractions need to be turned off while you talk with your children.) You love your children more than anyone, you care more than anyone, and they would rather hear from you first concerning any direct advice and answers you have about their questions on sexuality.

We parents can't get off the hook by simply explaining the "plumbing" or anatomy of the reproductive process or even the physical act of sex itself. Older teens are already likely to know at least some of that information and the books we select for our children can clarify any of those kinds of questions. Teens need detailed explanations about feelings and practical information to help them cope with unfamiliar emotions. No book written, that the authors are aware of, can tell your child as well as you can, what he or she needs to know concerning the strange new feelings they are experiencing. Seriously listening to your teen with sensitivity and a good sense of timing can be very helpful. We hope this book will be useful in answering some of the questions that may come up. You and your teen may want to read this book together. If you find yourself struggling for words when your child asks frank questions, take heart. You are not alone. Sometimes it feels like we are pioneers exploring new ground without a map to guide us. Congratulate yourself for having the courage to proceed into this new uncharted territory. Listen closely to your own inner feelings and memories as you guide your child.

There is a narrow space in time when we have the opportunity to give our children some of the best of us – our truths about feelings, what we'd like them to know about our basic beliefs, and facts to make life easier for them. We want to share with them our values such as integrity, justice, tolerance, hard work, good health, personal responsibility, loyalty and spirituality. We also want to make sure that they know certain skills, such as driving a car safely, buying and cooking healthy foods, how to write checks, and some polite ways to act at their grandparents' houses and other public places. We are, by definition, their mentors, their guides, and their rock in the storm.

We find ourselves worrying and asking:

- Will they know how to cope when they are first asked to experiment with sex in their peer group?
- Will they know how to protect themselves from disease and/or early pregnancy? And even if they know, will they **use** protection?
- Will they be able to recognize their feelings and act responsibly on them?
- Will they be able to communicate with caring adults and with their peers about what they really want and don't want?
- Will they have a good understanding (as a teen) of how difficult it is to be a parent and the wisdom to postpone parenthood until they have the maturity and the means to successfully support their child?

Those parents who, for whatever reason, have had the good fortune to build a trusting, open communication style with their child – the kind this book describes in earlier chapters -- are very lucky. They can talk with their children about such issues. For those who look back with regret at a less than happy relationship with a child, take heart. It is never too late to work on repairing damage already done, even though it is harder the later you start. It is **not** useful to point fingers or spend a lot of time feeling guilty over the past if your relationship with your child hasn't turned out the way you dreamed it could be. Remember, you did the best you could at the time. Many parents and grandparents have been able to reopen lines of communication with their young family members. All you really need is the will, the time and lots of patience along with some good information on human development. You may have had good communication with your young child only to find that, as a teen, he or she becomes silent and you may not know why. Keep talking with them in a friendly manner even if they refuse to respond. Silence from a parent is not recommended.

Children are very much aware of what you do and say whether **you** are aware of it or not.

Coming from homes where the "S" word was never mentioned, (much less any other helpful hints concerning sexuality), the authors, along with many other members of ours and past generations, have had to scramble to keep up with the "sexual revolution". We've had to struggle to learn how to give straight talk to our children and students. What a breath of fresh air it is to answer our children's questions simply and truthfully and watch them leave us with self-confidence, knowing that they have the tools to make sense of the complex world called "growing up". On the other hand, giving no information or false information to a questioning child is harmful to the child and to her/his relationship with you. When credibility is lost between a parent and child, time together can be full of pain and misunderstanding. If there is a problem, try to discuss it immediately.

Every question asked by your child about sex is asked sincerely even when it sounds like teasing. They expect straight answers from us. Stonewalling or treating the subject too lightly sends a negative message. Our children see their bodies and all their physiological functions as normal unless taught differently. We know that our U.S. culture has taught too many generations to be ashamed or overly titillated about their bodies and their sexuality. Today's youth look at matters of sexuality in a much more relaxed way than did their parents and grandparents. The Kaiser Foundation's research (1996) revealed that three-fourths of the teens asked felt that way. Many teens today see the whole realm of sexuality as "no big deal." They **do** want to know what's real and what works and doesn't work. Our fear is that they are becoming so relaxed about it all that they do not take health concerns seriously. The latest report from the Urban Institute published in December 2000, is that too many teens see non-coital sex as safe and therefore are not using protection for oral or anal sex. As parents we have to overcome our reluctance to discuss these topics and help our children stay safe.

The good news is that after 20 years of rising teen pregnancy rates, the numbers have begun to come down gradually. The National Center for Health Statistics reports that teens age 15 through 19, are having 48 births per 1000 teens. In 1997, it was double that figure (2001). What factors are responsible for this long hoped-for trend? Experts say that several factors are involved. The U.S. government and some state and private agencies are offering more courses and clinics for teens to receive information on responsible sex. Also, teens report that they are using

95

more condoms, injectable contraceptives and implants to prevent pregnancy. Reports show that even in programs that emphasize abstinence, information about safe sex is being taught. The non-partisan National Committee to Prevent Teen Pregnancy reports that the programs proven to be effective, using scientific measures, have been those that include information on both contraception and abstinence (*Newsweek*, 2000).

Not only are clinics and other programs offering more straight talk with teens but it is also likely that more parents are working up the courage to talk about sex and personal responsibility with their children **before** they grow into teenagers. If children feel that they can discuss these subjects with you, they can begin to think ahead about their responses to pushy peers who may try to tell them that all junior high kids should experience sex. You can point out that when children know they have choices, they can then feel that they have more control over their own bodies and can still have friends who respect them. Parents who begin conversation about these subjects early, usually find that their children avoid unwanted pregnancies later on. Too often, the subject isn't discussed until the teen is already pregnant.

Parenting Education for Teens

It is good to report that more and more parents today are recognizing the necessity of school classes offered to young teens to help them prepare for adulthood and, perhaps, parenthood. Teens want to hear from their parents about these serious issues but they also want to hear from teachers they respect. Then they can discuss what they are learning with their friends.

Statistics are showing that parenting education in schools can lessen violence in our society. Myrium Miedzian writes that boys respond to classes in childrearing that allow them to learn about caring for babies and families. They then feel more connected with others (Miedzian, 1991).

Nona Cannon, author of *ROOTS OF VIOLENCE, SEEDS OF PEACE*, says that "when people become more willing to educate themselves and their children for constructive family living, they will experience a reduction in many kinds of violence in families.... Family Life Education moves the world toward peace" (Cannon, 1996).

Since the 1960's, groups of active parents have struggled and won the right to have sex education classes in school districts scattered throughout the United States, often following verbal battles between school officials and other parents who believe in keeping the "S" word out of schools. We have discussed these objections previously in this book. Basically, the objections are based on values and beliefs that children are more likely to stay out of sexual trouble the less they know about the subject. We are talking about deep emotional beliefs where parents fail to see the strong statistical connection between increasingly effective sex education, parenting education and the reduction of teen pregnancies, not only in the United States, but in other developed countries whose track record is much better than ours.

Your Gift of Involvement as an Advocate for Our Children

Never doubt that a small group of thoughtful, committed citizens can change the world. Indeed, it's the only thing that has.

Margaret Mead

If you are convinced that our sons and daughters and grandchildren should be given quality classes in sex and parenting education in junior and senior high schools, then we have to take a big step forward and join with others to move closer to this goal. Changes in public school policies are made when like-minded citizens come together to express their wishes to local, state and federal lawmakers. The lawmakers may vote for the monies needed if we work as organized political lobbyists for our cause.

The word "political" can bring up negative reactions in many of us. Granted, if we have not had any experience working for honest politicians, (and there are many) it is hard to have faith in the political system. The old saying that "our lawmakers are only as good as those who vote them in" is all too true. When we ignore the political system and fail to exercise our power to shape public policy as we believe it should be, then we ignore the reality of how laws are passed. Most citizens get tired of pushing for change in government and give up. Unscrupulous politicians count on us bowing out. But honest politicians hope we will be persistent by assisting and supporting them in their efforts to improve our institutions. When we become active in our political system, our children watch how we work to make a difference. They learn from our actions that it **is** possible to make changes in society if we follow a few proven guidelines.

97

As community activists for 40 years, the authors have learned that when an individual joins forces with a group of like-minded citizens, amazing results are achieved. Whether you choose to lead a group or become an active member of one, your energy, combined with others, is what will help produce the kind of changes you are after. For those of us who are especially interested in creating more sex education and parenting education classes, it is important to contact those organizations which have already been actively working for these goals. They have valuable information on the most effective organizational tools. Appendix C lists a number of such groups.

One highly successful lobbying group is the California Association for the Education of Young Children (CAEYC), an affiliate of the National Association for the Education of Young Children. This California group has published *A RESOURCE GUIDE: CHILD ADVOCACY IN 10 EASY STEPS* (Pearce, 1988). This guide advises that, as budding political activists, we should identify which problems are most important to us and inspire us to action. That action might be a call to a legislator or to join a like-minded group. Taking immediate action is most effective if you do your homework and find out who is already working on your particular concern, what has already been done about the problem and where you can offer the help that is most needed. If you don't know anyone who is already working on your concern, call an organization and request their materials or call your lawmaker's office for guidance.

The Children's Defense Fund (CDF), a leading national advocacy group founded by its President, Marion Wright Edelman, has led the fight for children's rights and is responsible, in coalition with other groups, for changing much of the legislative landscape on behalf of children. Mrs. Edelman has been active in supporting the movement for parenting education in the schools as well. Each year CDF publishes *THE STATE OF AMERICA'S CHILDREN* to make us aware of the tremendous needs of America's youth (CDF, 2001). In Mrs. Edelman's words, "As an American community [we] commit ourselves to putting you, our children first, to building a just America that leaves no child behind, and to ensuring all of you a healthy and safe passage to adulthood" (Edelman, 1998).

The Parenting Project, a national organization dedicated to furthering parenting education in the schools is another excellent group (see Appendix C) to contact. They have provided effective leadership in convincing a number of school districts that parenting education is needed for our young teens. At this writing there is no state where parenting education is mandated for all junior and senior high schools. One of California's finest legislators, Senator John Vasconcellos, has dedicated his energies for the last eight years to passing a state mandated parenting education bill only to have it vetoed by California governors. The bill made provisions for giving students positive learning experiences in the classroom in such areas as personal hygiene, parental responsibility, multiple life skills, self-esteem, teen parenting issues, child development, child abuse, good communication and maintaining healthy relationships (Vasconcellos, 2000).

Other states attempting to pass such a bill find that objections come from their legislatures, Boards of Education or School Superintendents. Teens can enroll in cooking classes and car mechanics in almost any school district, yet are being denied the opportunity to discover skills to help them be better adults and parents. We, as a country, would never allow medical information to be withheld from our children, and yet many parents and officials still stand by and allow critical information to be withheld, perhaps with the hope that the children will learn all they need to know at home. The statistics on unwanted pregnancies and the rise in sexually transmitted disease infections refute that kind of wishful thinking (Children's Defense Fund, 2001). In 1996, Mary Fisher, an AIDs victim, appeared on a television interview and shared these words, "If we don't tell them what we know about protection from HIV, then we're not loving them very much." At the Republican National Convention in 1992, she spoke these words, "If you do not see this killer stalking your children, look again." Her speech ended with an appeal for education: "Learn with me the lessons of history and of grace, so my children will not be afraid to say the word AIDS when I am gone. Then their children and yours, may not need to whisper it at all."

In all our years of college teaching, we have yet to meet a student who disagrees with the idea of offering quality parenting education in junior and senior high school classes. Although they often complain that they get too little information in the classes they have taken. They also want to know where they can learn the principles of child development without becoming a psychology or early childhood education major. Their cry for help is very real. The time for parenting education classes in our schools is now! Even presidential candidates during the 2000 campaign mentioned the need for this kind of education. Just as we are dedicated to helping our children better understand their sexuality and the importance of responsibility for their actions, let us work to be sure that all children receive reliable and honest information in their school classes as well.

Our children watch and wait for us to find the courage to shape a better world for them than the one we have known. As pioneers, the way is never easy -- but with love, all things are possible.

ABOUT THE AUTHORS

JANE CARNEY SCHULZE, Ph.D. is a faculty member in Sociology at San Diego State University, Department of Sociology, and Southwestern College in the Department of Child Development. She has been a teacher in preschools through college for the past 43 years. She has counseled diverse families with children of all ages and consulted with various programs such as Head Start, the California Council on Wellness and Physical Fitness, the YMCA and public and private schools. She co-founded two preschools for children with emotional-behavioral problems, working with the community, parents, and professionals. She has written and spoken extensively on family issues in the U.S. as well as internationally, and was named North American Coordinator for the United Nations' International Year of the Family, 1994. She continues to be active in promoting Parenting Education classes in public and private schools. She and her husband, Rolf, reside in San Diego, California, where they enjoy quality time with their children and grandchildren.

ROLF SCHULZE, Ph.D., Professor Emeritus of Sociology at San Diego State University, pioneered a course in Human Sexuality in the Department of Sociology in the early 1970's, which he continued to teach for 25 years. He has published in the area of Sexuality, Social Psychology, and Political Sociology. He continues to teach a popular course in Contemporary Social Problems and is active in the community. He has extensive international experience, having both lived, studied, lectured, and researched abroad.

ACKNOWLEDGEMENTS

This book is a composite of our learning experiences with many people who are important in our lives. Our students, preschool through college age, with whom we have worked over a 40-year span, our friends and colleagues and our children and grandchildren, have all helped us learn better ways to communicate with them.

This work would never have reached print without the guidance of Roland Summit, community psychiatrist at Harbor/UCLA Medical Center from 1966 to 1999. His editing and experienced perspectives in this field added immeasurably to the book.

Our dear friend and colleague, Nona Cannon, Professor Emerita, San Diego State University in Family Studies, gave invaluable input to the manuscript for which we are most grateful. Her lifelong leadership on developing peaceful humans has been our ongoing inspiration.

Rena Wallace, tireless editor and creative designer, has added greatly to the presentation and artistic layout of this book and transformed it into the finished product. Thanks also to our nephew, Chuck Wallace, and our daughter Amara Karuna, who provided the chapter illustrations.

We especially thank our children, Mark, Eric, Bonnie, Dan and Amara for encouraging us to pursue this project and for offering their wise advice on many issues. We have learned much from them.

To our grandchildren, Guy Peter, Jason, Ryan, Russell and Heron, thank you for being our friends and letting us quote you!

Grateful appreciation goes to our brother, Chuck Wallace, anthropologist, who has never settled for less than the best in his life and works. He constantly encourages us to learn, to write and to become more aware.

And finally, we are grateful to all of those who have, over the years, helped to further our education and learning about what it means to become full human beings. We hope all of our efforts will make a difference to those who read this book.

Jane Carney Schulze and Rolf Schulze

REFERENCES

Allen, L., *et al.* (1991). The Effects of Intrauterine Cocaine Exposure: Transient or Teratogenic? *Archives of Clinical Neurospsychology*, 6, 133-146.

Baby Think It Over, (1999). BTIO, Educational Products, Inc., 2709 Mondovi, Eau Claire, WI, 54701.

Barovick, H. (1998, June 15). Dr. Drew, After Hours Guru. *Time*.

Baruch, D. (1959). New Ways in Sex Education. NY: McGraw-Hill.

Bell, R. (1998). Changing Bodies, Changing Lives. NY: Random House.

Berk, L. (2002). Infants, Children and Adolescents. Boston: Allyn & Bacon.

Berns, R. (1998) Child, Family, Community. Fort Worth: Harcourt Brace College Publishers.

Cannon, N. (1996). Roots of Violence, Seeds of Peace in People, Families and Society. San Diego: Miclearoy Publishing.

Carns, D. (1973) Talking About Sex: Notes on First Coitis and Double Sexual Standard. *Journal of Marriage and the Family*, 35, 677-688.

Children's Defense Fund (1987). Adolescent Pregnancy: An Anatomy of a Social Problem in Search of Comprehensive Solutions. Washington, D.C.: Children's Defense Fund.

Children's Defense Fund, (2001). The State of America's Children, 2001. Washington, D.C.: Children's Defense Fund.
Circulo de Hombres, (1998). Logan Heights Family Health Center brochure. San Diego: 2204 National Ave., San Diego, CA, 92113.

Comer, J. (1998). in Berns, R., Child, Family, School Community. Ft. Worth: Harcourt Brace College Publishers.
Comstock G., and Paik, H. (1991). Television and the American Child. San Diego: Academic Press.

Conger L. (1977). Adolescence and Youth. New York: Harper and Row.

Daniels, S. (2001, October, 14). Teens Sitting in the Driver's Seat. *San Diego Union Tribune*, E-4.

DeSisto, P. (1996, November 24). Intervention for Violent Adolescents www.teachersworkshop.com. Cooperative Discipline Institute.

Edelman, M. (1998). Stand for Children. New York: Hyperion Books for Children.

Erikson, E. (1982). The Life Cycle Completed. New York: Norton.

Erikson, E. (1963). Childhood and Society. New York: Norton.

Faber, A., and Mazlish, E. (1980). How to Talk So Kids Will Listen, and Listen So Kids Will Talk. New York: Avon Books.

Gagnon, J., and Simon, W. (1973). Sexual Conduct: The Social Sources of Human Sexuality. Chicago: Aldine Publishing Company.

Gardner, H. (1983). Frames of Mind: The Theory of Multiple Intelligences. New York: Basic Books.
Gerrard, M. (1987). Sex, Guilt, and Contraceptive Use Revisited: The 1980's. *Journal of Personality and Social Psychology*, 52, 975-980.
Ginott, H. (1969). Parent and Teenager. New York: The MacMillan Company.

Goldhagen, S. (2001, September). Let's Talk About Sex. *Teenstyle*. 42-46.

Gordon, T. (1970). Parent Effectiveness Training. New York: Peter H. Wyden.

Green, R. (1980). Homosexuality, in H. Kaplan, A. Freedman, and B.Sadock (Eds.). Comprehensive Textbook of Psychiatry. (Vol. 2) (3rd ed.). Baltimore: Williams and Wilkins.

Green, R. (1987). The "Sissy Boy" Syndrome and the Development of Homosexuality. New Haven: Yale University Press.

Goldstein, A. (2000, July 3). Paging All Parents. *Time*, p.47.

Gunn, R. M.D. (1996, Sept. 8). Letter to the Editor. *San Diego Union Tribune*.

Guttmacher, A. (1997). Alan Guttmacher Institute: Center for Disease Control and Prevention. 120 Wall Street, New York, N.Y. 10005

Hackbert, W. (In Press). The Good Book.

Hannaford, C. (1987, February 5). *Germantown News*, p. 1.

Hatcher, R. *et al.* (1996). Contraceptive Technology. New York: Irvington Publishers.

Hendrick, J. (1990). Total Learning. New York: McMillan College Publishing Company.
Hildebrand, V. (2000). Parenting, Rewards and Responsibilities. New York: Glencoe McGraw-Hill.

Hite, S. (1995, June). Secrets Mothers Keep. *New Woman*, 96-99.

Intermountain Health Care. (1993). Building Your Family Dream. Salt Lake City: National Association of Counties.

Jones, E., *et al.* (1987). Teenage Pregnancy in Industrialized Countries. New Haven: Yale University Press.

Kaiser Family Foundation. (1996, June 25). Teens Want More Information on Birth Control. Princeton Research Survey, March 1996. *San Diego Union Tribune*. A-1.

Kaiser Family Foundation. (1996). Talking With Kids About Tough Issues. Hotline: (800) CHILD-44.

Kinsey, A., Pomeroy, E., and Martin, C. (1948). Sexual Behavior in the Human Male. Philadelphia: Saunders.

Kinsey, A., *et al.* (1953) Sexual Behavior in the Human Female. Philadelphia: Saunders Publishing Company.

Louv, R., (1996, August 25). On Matters of Sex, Teens Are Ready to Listen. Roper Starch Survey. *San Diego Union Tribune*, E-1.

Malina, R., and Bouchard, C. (1991). Growth, Maturation, and Physical Activity. Champaign, Illinois: Human Kinetics.

McCord, J. (1991). Questioning the Value of Punishment. Social Problems. 38: 167-179.

McMahon, T. (1996, December 7). Teen tips, a survival guide for parents with kids 11 through 19. Pocket Books. Reported in San Diego Union: Primer on youth is for and by parents, E-5.

Mead, M. (1974). Speech given at The First Unitarian-Universalist Church, San Diego, California.

Michael, R.T., *et al.* (1994). Sex in America. Boston: Little, Brown

Miedzian, M. (1991). Boys Will be Boys. New York: Doubleday.

Miller, K., Levin, M., Whitaker, D., and Xu, X. (1998). Patterns of Condom Use Among Adolescents. The Impact of Mother-Adolescent Communication. *American Journal of Public Health*, 88, 1542-1544.

Napier, C. (1996). The Power of Abstinence. Fairfield, New Jersey: Morrow, William and Company.

National Center for Health Statistics. (2000). Center for Disease Control and Prevention. 6525 Belcrest Road, Rm. 1064, Hyattsville, Maryland, 20782.
National Center for Health Statistics. (2000). News Release. www.cdc.gov

National Center on Addiction and Drug Abuse. (1999). Columbia University, New York, N.Y.

Newsweek (2000, May 8). The Naked Truth. 58-59.

Papalia, D., and Olds, S. (1996). A Child's World: Infancy Through Adolescence. New York: McGraw-Hill.

Papp, L. (1999, January 23). Family Ties Can Help Avoid Teen Pregnancy. *The Toronto Star.*

Pearce, M. (1988). Child Advocacy in 10 Easy Steps, A Resource Guide. Sacramento: California Association for the Education of Young Children. Peraino, J. *et al.* (1998). Program Evaluation of the 4th Through 6th Grades. Spanish Primary Prevention Program. Houston Advocates for Mental health in Children.

Pipher, M. (1994). Reviving Ophelia. New York: Ballantine Books.

Planned Parenthood, (1998). Fact Sheets: Helping Young People to Delay Sexual Intercourse. www.plannedparenthood.org

Prescott, J. (1975, April). Body Pleasure and the Origins of Violence. *The Futurist*, 64-74.

Reynolds, E. (1996). Guiding Young Children, A Problem Solving Approach. Mountain View, California: Mayfield Publishing.

Santelli, J. M.D. (1998, June 15). Where'd You Learn That? *Time.*

Savin-Williams, R. (1988). Theoretical Perspectives Accounting for Homosexuality. *Journal of Adolescent Health Care*, 9, 95-104.

Sorensen, R. (1973). Adolescent Sexuality in Contemporary Society. New York: World Book.
Spock, B. (1998). The Common Sense Book of Baby and Child Care. New York: Pocket Books.

Steinberg, L. (1993). Adolescence. New York: McGraw-Hill.

Summit, R. (1983). The Child Sexual Abuse Accommodation Syndrome. *Child Abuse And Neglect*, 7:177-193.

Summit, R. (1990). Abuse of the Child Sexual Abuse Accommodation Syndrome. *Journal of Child Sexual Abuse*, 4:153-163.

Swets, P. (1995). The Art of Talking With Your Teenagers. Holbrook, Maine: Adams Media.

Tanner, J. (1990). Foetus Into Man. Cambridge, Massachusetts: Harvard University Press.

Tyree, C. et al. (1991, March). Restructuring the Public School Curriculum to Include Parenting Education Classes. Paper presented at the annual meeting of the Southern Association on Children Under 6. Atlanta.

Urban Institute. (2000. December). Urban Institute Report.

Vasconcellos, J. (2000). California State Senate Bill 1348. Introducing mandatory parenting education classes into junior high and high schools.

Wallis, C. (1999, July 5). The Kids Are Alright. *Time*, 56-58.

Westheimer, R. (1998). Dr. Ruth Talks to Kids. Old Tappan, New Jersey: Simon and Schuster Children Books.

Westoff, C. (1988). Unintended Pregnancy in America and Abroad. *Family Planning Perspectives*, 20, 254-261.

White House Conference on Children and Youth. (1997) Washington, D.C.

Wingert, P. (1998, May 11). The Battle Over Falling Birthrates. *Newsweek*. Wolf, R. (1996). Marriages and Families in a Diverse Society. New York: Harper Collins Publishers.

APPENDIXES

Appendix A: Information for Parents of Newborns Through Adolescence

Apter, T. (1990). Altered Loves: Mothers and Daughters During Adolescence. New York: St. Martin's.

How mother and daughter relationships change.

Baby Think It Over, Inc., 2709 Mondovi Road. Eau Claire, Wisconsin, 54701. (800) 830-1416.

An infant simulator for teens to practice infant care at home and in the classroom.

Bell, Ruth (1998). Changing Bodies, Changing Lives. New York: Random House.

An excellent reference for young teens to help them understand what is happening to their bodies.

Cannon, Nona (1996). Roots of Violence, Seeds of Peace in People, Families and Society. Maclieory Press: San Diego.

The author's concept of "Self-Otherness" would help us live in a more peaceful world.

Child Help USA, Inc., www.childhelpusa.org. Hotline: 1-800-4-A-CHILD.

Enables parents to request information or speak to a crisis counselor.

De Toledo, Sylvia, and Deborah Brown (1995). Grandparents As Parents, a Survival Guide for Raising a Second Family. New York: Guilford Press.

Ginott, Haim (1969). Between Parent and Teenager. New York: MacMillan.

Glennon, Will (2000). 200 Ways to Raise a Boy's Emotional Intelligence. Berkeley: Conari Press.

Glennon, Will (1999) 200 Ways to Raise a Girl's Self Esteem. Berkeley: Conari Press.

Grandparents Raising Grandchildren Organization. P.O. Box 104, Colleyville, Texas, 76034. (817) 577-0435.

Offers emotional support.

Hildebrand, Verna (2000). Parenting: Rewards and Responsibilities. Teachers' classroom resources including a text for parenting education classes. Peoria, Illinois: Glencoe/McGraw-Hill.

Leach, Penelope (1990). Your Baby and Child From Birth to Age 5. New York: Knopf.

Comprehensive guide for child's first five years of life.

McCoy, K., and Wibblesman, C. (1992). The New Teenage Body Book. New York: Putman.

Describes what happens as teens mature, balancing emotional and sexual sides of growing up.

Miedzian, Myriam (1991). Boys Will Be Boys: Breaking the Link Between Masculinity and Violence. New York: Doubleday.

Provides a useful description of effective programs to help boys learn empathy on their way to becoming nurturing fathers.

Montagu, Ashley (1971). Touching. New York: Columbia University Press.

Pipher, Mary (1994). Reviving Ophelia: Saving the Selves of Adolescent Girls. New York: Ballantine Books.

Pipher, Mary (1996). The Shelter of Each Other, Rebuilding Our Families. New York: Random House.

Planned Parenthood Federation of America, Sexual Health Resources Catalog. 810 Seventh Ave. New York: NY 10019. 1-800-669-0156.

Planned Parenthood Federation of America (1996) Talking About Sex, A Guide for Families. Marketing Dept., Planned Parenthood of America, 810 Seventh Ave. New York, NY 10019. 1-800-669-0156.

Includes a cartoon format video and booklet to help families answer their children's questions about sexual matters including puberty, anatomy, sexual orientation, birth control, pregnancy, sexually transmitted diseases and sexual abuse.

Poe, Lenora (1992). Black Grandparents As Parents. 2034 Blake St., Berkeley, California

Steinberg, Laurence, and Ann Levine (1990). You and Your Adolescent: A Parent's Guide For Ages 10-20. New York: Harper Collins.

Helping parents with questions on most adolescent issues.

Swets, Paul (1995). The Art of Talking With Your Teenager. Holbrook, MA: Adams Media.

Sex Education, Teen Pregnancy and Parenting Catalog. Nimco: PO Box 9, 102 Highway 81 N, Calhoun, KY 42327-0009. 1-800-962-6662.

United States Centers for Disease Control, www.cdc.gov.

Government agency devoted to promoting health and controlling diseases. Disseminates information. Sponsors the National AIDS Hotline: 1-800-342-AIDS and the National STD Hotline: 1-800-227-8922.

APPENDIX B: CHILDREN'S BOOKS

Avery, Charles (1992). Everybody Has Feelings: Todos Tenemos Sentimientos: The Moods of Children. Beltsville, Maryland: Gryphon House.

For children and preteens.

Brandenburg, Aliki (1984). Feelings. New York: Mulberry Books/William Morrow.

Preschool level.

Brown, Laurie, and Marc Brown. (1997). What's The Big Secret? Talking About Sex with Girls and Boys. Boston: Little, Brown and Co.

Anatomy, feelings, sex and pregnancy discussions for older children and preteens.

Cole, Joanna. (1984). How You Were Born. New York: William Morrow.

Large photo illustrations for preschoolers.

Cole, Joanna (2001). When You Were Inside Mommy. New York: Harper Collins.

> *For preschoolers.*

Coombs, Samm (1977). Teenage Survival Manual; Why Parents Act That Way and Other Mysteries of Mind and Matter. San Francisco: Halo Books.

Corwin, Donna (1999). The Tween Years; A Parent's Guide for Surviving Those Terrific, Turbulent, and Trying Times Between Childhood and Adolescence. Chicago: NTC Contemporary Publishing Group.

Davis, Jennifer (2001). First Comes Love: All About the Birds and the Bees and Alligators, Possums, and People, Too. New York: Workman Publishing.

> *For older children / pre-teens.*

Ezzo, Gary and Robert Bucknam, M.D., (2000). On Becoming Teenwise. Sisters, Oregon: Mutnomakh Publishers.

Harris, Robie (1994). It's Perfectly Normal, Changing bodies, Growing Up, Sex and Sexual Health. Cambridge: Candlewick Press.

> *From conception and puberty to birth control and AIDS.*

Harris, Robie (1999). It's So Amazing! A book About Eggs, Sperm, Birth, Babies and Families. Cambridge: Candlewick Press.

Ingoglia, Gina (1989), Look Inside Your Body. New York: Grosset and Dunlap.

> *Preschool age.*

Jakes, Mavis (1998). Growing Up, It's a Girl Thing. New York: Alfred A. Knopf.

> *Straight talk about first bras, first periods, and changing bodies.*

Madares, Lynda, with Area Madares (2000). The What's Happening to My Body? Book for Girls: A Growing Up Guide for Parents and Daughters. New York: Newmarket Press.

Madares, Lynda, and Madares, Area (2000). The What's Happening to My Body? Book for Boys: A Growing Up Guide for Parents and Sons. New York: Newmarket Press.

Marcus, Eric (2000). What IF Someone I Know Is Gay? Answers to Questions About Gays and Lesbian People. New York: Penguin Putnam Books for Young Readers.

Mayle, Peter (1975). What's Happening to Me? New York: Kensington Publishing Corporation.

Explaining puberty to children.

Mayle, Peter (1977). Where Did I Come From? African American Edition (2000). New York: Kensington Publishing.

The facts of life for children. Humorous illustrations.

Murkoff, Heidi (2000). What to Expect When Mommy's Having A Baby. New York: Harper Collins.

Pogany Susan (1998). Sex Smart, 501 Reasons to Hold Off On Sex. Minneapolis: Fairview Press.

For young teens.

Potash, Marlin, and Laura Frutman (2001). Am I Weird Or Is This Normal? Advice and Information to Get Teens in the Know. New York: Simon and Schuster.

Pruett, Kyle (1999). Me, Myself and I. How Children Build Their Sense of Self, 18 to 36 Months. New York: Goddard Press.

Schaefer, Valerie (1998). The Care and Keeping of You: The Body Book for Girls. American Girl Library Editor. Pleasant Company Publications, 8400 Fairway Place, PO Box 620998 Middleton, Wisconsin 53562.

Wachter, Oralee (1983). No More Secrets For Me. A Book for Adults to Share with Children. New York: O.D.N. Productions.

Sexual abuse is a secret no child should have to keep.

Waxman, Stephanie (1976). What Is A Girl? What Is A Boy? Culver City: Peace Press.

For young children / pre-teens.

APPENDIX C: ADVOCACY INFORMATION FOR FAMILIES AND THEIR CHILDREN

Association for Childhood Education International (AECI) 17904 Georgia Ave. Ste. 215, Olney, MD 20832.

Blank, Helen, and Poersch, Nicole (1996). Working With State and Local Officials: A Guide for Early Care and Educational Advocates. Children's Defense Fund, 25 E St. NW, Washington, DC 2001.

Children's Defense Fund 25 E St. NW, Washington, DC 2001.

Dedicated to "Leave No Child Behind." Promotes legislation to give all children in the United States a good start. Publishes numerous research findings on poverty and its consequences in the United States.

National Association for the Education of Young Children, (NAEYC).

1509 16th St. NW, Washington, DC 20036-1426.

Broad spectrum of services for teachers who work with young children and parents. Publishes a professional journal with the latest research on child care and development.

The Parenting Project. Preparing tomorrow's parents today. A national advocacy group supporting the efforts of parents and educators to put parenting education classes in schools. 5776 Hamilton Way Boca Raton, Florida 33496 1-888-PARENTS.

Pearce, Marilyn (1988). Child Advocacy in 10 Easy Steps: A Resource Guide. California Association for the Education of Young Children (CAEYC). P.O. Box 160373, Sacramento, CA 95816.

Details on how to be effective for children's issues within the political system.

Pozmantier, Jan (1996). Teaching Children Today The Parenting Skills They Will Need Tomorrow. Primary Prevention Program of Houston Advisory for Mental Health in Children. 6209 Skyline, Houston, Texas 77057.

National Council on Child Abuse and Family Violence, 1155 Connecticut Ave. NW, Ste. 300, Washington, DC 20036. (202) 429-6695.

Schwartz, Pepper, and Dominic Cappello (2000). Ten Talks Parents Must Have With Their Children About Sex and Character. New York: Hyperion.

Spock, Benjamin (2001) Martin T. Stein, Editor. Dr. Spock's The School Years: The Emotional and Social Development of Children. New York: Pocket Books.

Made in the USA
Lexington, KY
30 May 2015